JOHN BERGER
A Fortunate Man

John Berger was born in London in 1926. He is well known for his novels and stories as well as for his works of nonfiction, including several volumes of art criticism. His first novel, *A Painter of Our Time*, was published in 1958, and since then his books have included the novel *G.*, which won the Booker Prize in 1972, and the peasant trilogy *Into Their Labours*, which includes *Pig Earth* (1979), *Once in Europa* (1987), and *Lilac and Flag* (1990). His six volumes of essays include *Keeping a Rendezvous* (1991), *The Sense of Sight* (1985), and *Ways of Seeing* (1972). In 1962 Berger left Britain permanently, and he now lives in a small village in the French Alps.

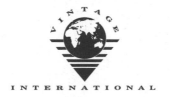

INTERNATIONAL

ALSO BY JOHN BERGER

To the Wedding

Into Their Labours
(Pig Earth, Once in Europa, Lilac and Flag: A Trilogy)

A Painter of Our Time

Permanent Red

The Foot of Clive

Corker's Freedom

Art and Revolution

The Moment of Cubism and Other Essays

The Look of Things: Selected Essays and Articles

Ways of Seeing

Another Way of Telling

A Seventh Man

G.

About Looking

And Our Faces, My Heart, Brief as Photos

Keeping a Rendezvous

A

FORTUNATE

MAN

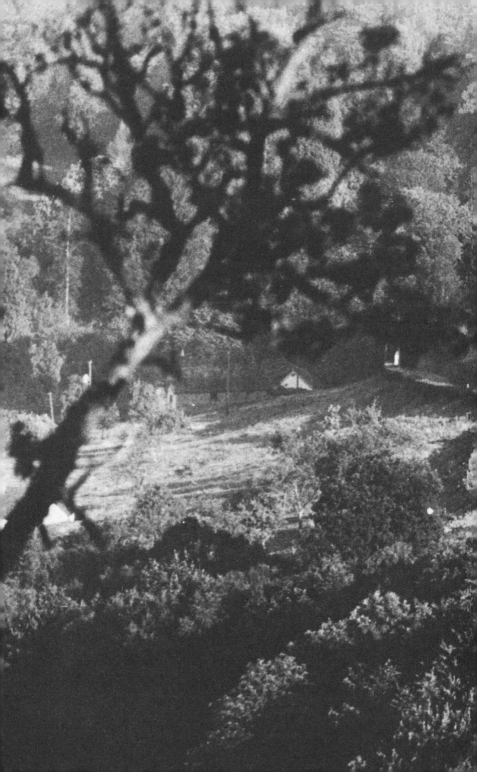

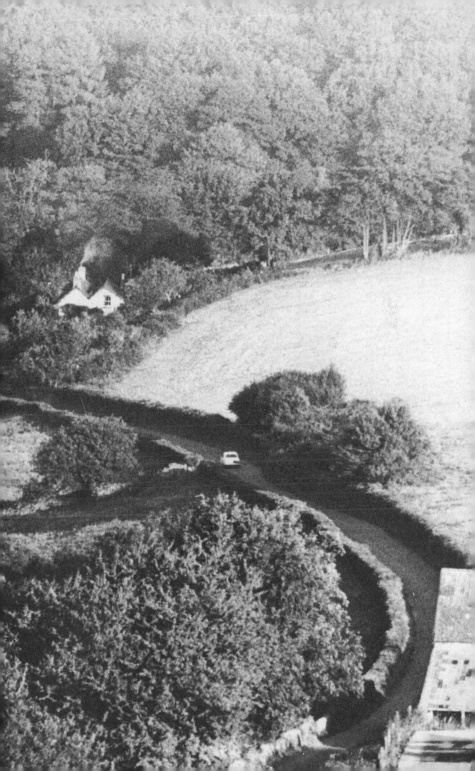

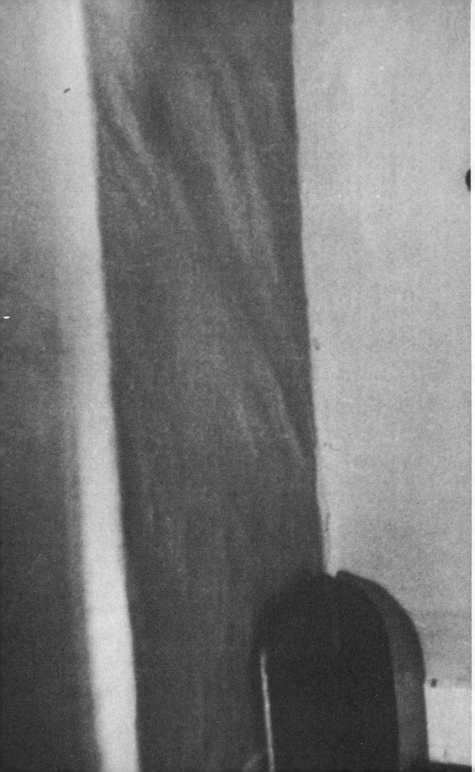

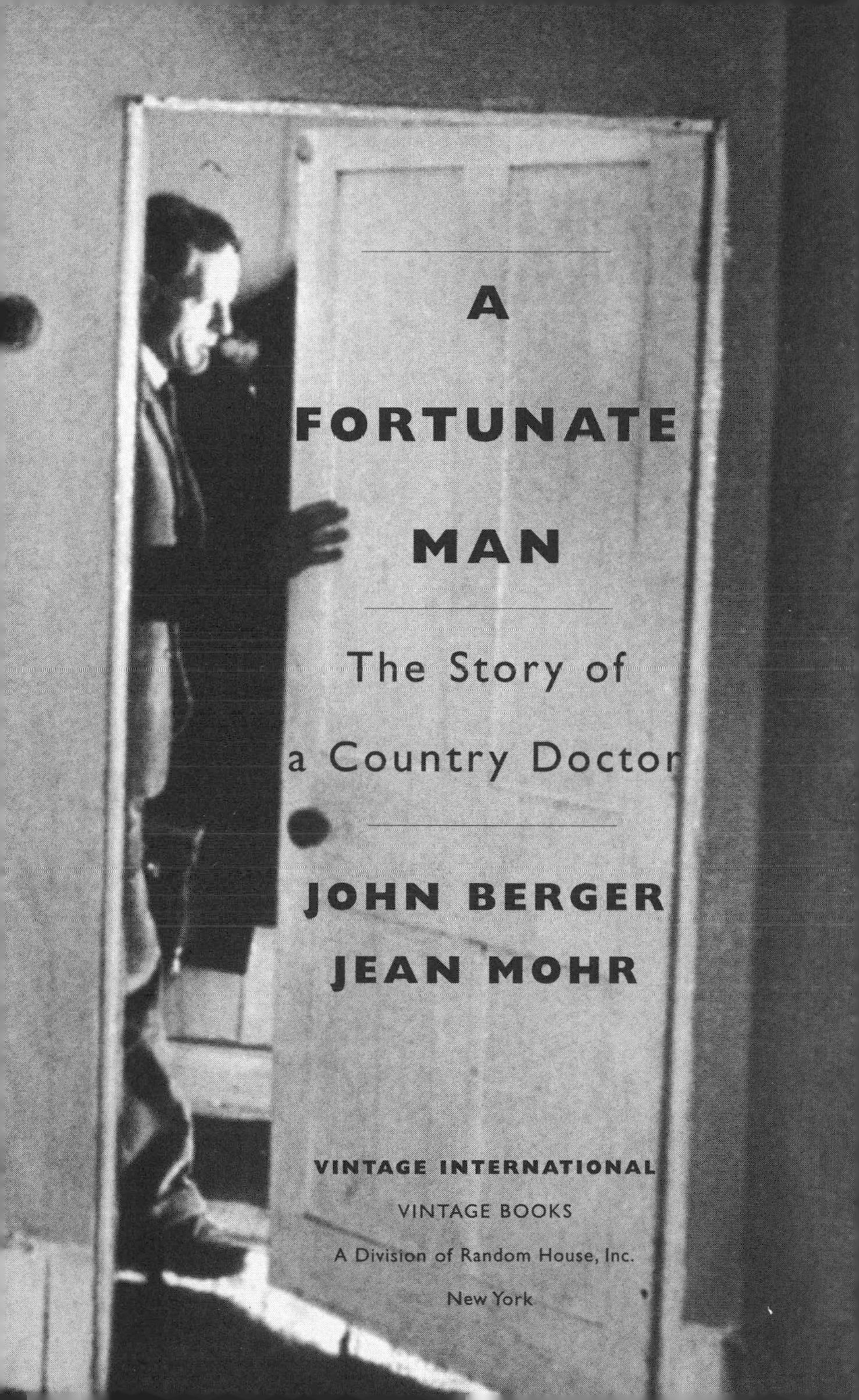

A

FORTUNATE

MAN

The Story of
a Country Doctor

JOHN BERGER
JEAN MOHR

VINTAGE INTERNATIONAL

VINTAGE BOOKS

A Division of Random House, Inc.

New York

First Vintage International Edition, February 1997

The Library of Congress has cataloged the Pantheon edition as follows:

Berger, John, [date]
A fortunate man / John Berger : photographs by Jean Mohr.
p. cm.
ISBN 0-394-73999-X
1. Sassall, John. 2. Physicians (General practice)—England—Biography.
3. Medicine, Rural—England
I. Mohr, Jean. II. Title.
R489.S2B4 1981
610'.92'4 [B]
81-47187
CIP

Vintage ISBN: 0-679-73726-X

Random House Web address: http://www.randomhouse.com/

Printed in the United States of America
10

This book is dedicated
to John and Betty whom it concerns, and
to Philip O'Connor
for the letters he wrote to me whilst I was writing it.
J.B.

A

FORTUNATE

MAN

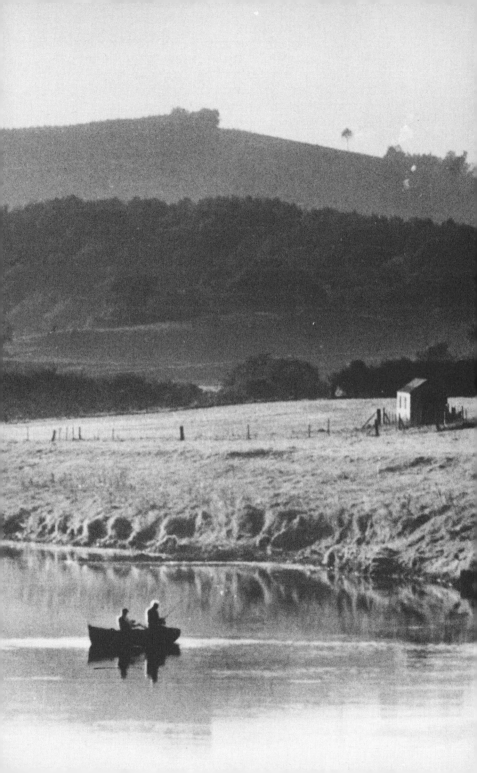

Landscapes can be deceptive.
Sometimes a landscape seems to be less a setting
for the life of its inhabitants than a curtain behind which
their struggles, achievements and accidents take place.

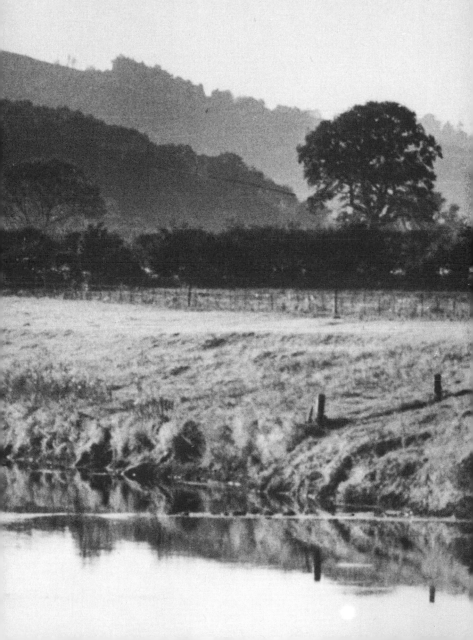

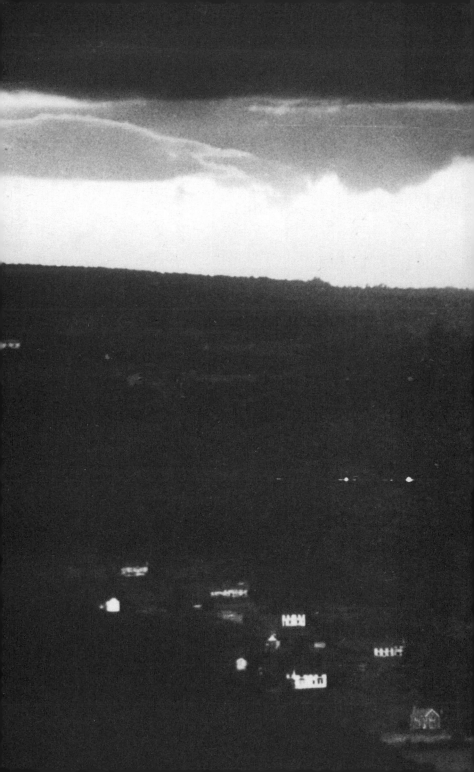

For those who, with the inhabitants, are behind
the curtain, landmarks are no longer only geographic
but also biographical and personal.

One of them shouted a warning, but it was too late. The leaves brushed him down almost delicately. The small branches encaged him. And then the tree and the whole hill crushed him together.

A man breathlessly said that a woodman was trapped beneath a tree. The doctor asked the dispenser to find out exactly where: then suddenly picked up his own phone, interrupted her and spoke himself. He must know exactly where. Which was the nearest gate in the nearest field? Whose field? He would need a stretcher. His own stretcher had been left in hospital the day before. He told the dispenser to phone immediately for an ambulance and tell it to wait by the bridge which was the nearest point on the road. At home in the garage there was an old door off its hinges. Blood plasma from the dispensary, door from the garage. As he drove through the lanes he kept his thumb on the horn the whole time, partly to warn oncoming traffic, partly so that the man under the tree might hear it and know that the doctor was coming.

After five minutes he turned off the road and drove uphill, into the mist. As often up there above the river, it was a very white mist, a mist that seemed to deny all weight and solidity. He had to stop twice to open gates. The third gate was already slightly open, so he drove through it without stopping. It swung back and crashed against the rear of the Land Rover. Some sheep, startled, appeared and disappeared into the mist. All the while he had his thumb on the horn for the woodman to hear. After one more field he saw a figure waving behind the mist – as if he were try-ing to wipe clean a vast steamed-up window.

When the doctor reached him the man said: 'He's been screaming ever since. He's suffering some-thing terrible doctor.' The man would tell the story many times, and the first would be tonight in the

village. But it was not yet a story. The advent
of the doctor brought the conclusion much nearer, but
the accident was not yet over: the wounded man
was still screaming at the other two men who
were hammering in wedges preparatory to lifting the tree.

'Christ let me alone.' As he cried 'alone' the doctor
was beside him. The wounded man recognized the
doctor; his eyes focused. For him too the conclusion was
nearer and this gave him the courage to be quieter.
Suddenly it was silent. The men had stopped
hammering but were still kneeling on the ground. They
knelt and looked at the doctor. His hands are at
home on a body. Even these new wounds which had
not existed twenty minutes before were familiar to
him. Within seconds of being beside the man he injected
morphine. The three onlookers were
relieved by the doctor's presence. But now his very
sureness made it seem to them that he was part of the
accident: almost its accomplice.

'He had a chance,' said one of the kneeling men,
'when Harry here shouted but he went and turned about
the wrong way.'

The doctor set up the plasma for a transfusion into
the arm. As he moved around, he explained what
he was doing to try to reassure the others.

'I shouted at him,' said Harry, 'he could have got
clear if he'd looked sharp.'

'He would have got clear like that,' said the third.

As the morphine worked, the wounded man's
face relaxed and his eyes closed. It was then as though
the relief he felt was so intense that it reached the
others.

'He's lucky to be alive,' said Harry.

'He could have got clear like that,' said the third.

The doctor asked them if they could shift the tree.

'I reckon we can if we are three now.'

Nobody was kneeling any longer. The three woods-
men were standing, impatient to begin. The mist
was getting whiter. The moisture was condensing on

the half-empty bottle of plasma. The doctor noticed
that this fractionally changed its colour, making it look
yellower than normal.

'I want you to lift,' he said, 'while I put a splint on
his leg.'

When the wounded man felt the reverberations in the
tree as they levered it, he began to moan again.

'We could injure him worse than ever,' said Harry,
'getting him out.' He could see the crushed
leg underneath like a dog killed on the road.

'Just hold it steady,' said the doctor.

Again the doctor, whom they knew so well, seemed
the accomplice of disaster as he worked under the
tree on the leg the fourth of them would lose.

'We'd never believed you'd got here so quick, doc,'
said the third.

'You know Sleepy Joe?' asked the doctor. 'He was
trapped under a tree for twelve hours before any
help came.'

He gave instructions on how to lift the wounded man
on to the door and then into the back of the Land
Rover.

'You'll be all right now Jack,' said one of them to the
wounded man whose face was as damp and pallid as
the mist. The third touched his shoulder.

The ambulance was waiting at the bridge. When it had
driven off, Harry turned to the doctor confidentially.

'He's lost his leg,' he said, 'hasn't he?'

'No, he won't lose his leg,' said the doctor.

The woodman walked slowly back up to the forest.
As he climbed he put a hand on each thigh. He told
the other two what the doctor had told him. As they
worked there during the day stripping the tree,
they noticed again and again the hollow in the ground
where he had been trapped. The fallen leaves there
were so dark and wet that it was impossible to
distinguish the blood. But every time they noticed the
place they questioned whether the doctor could
be right.

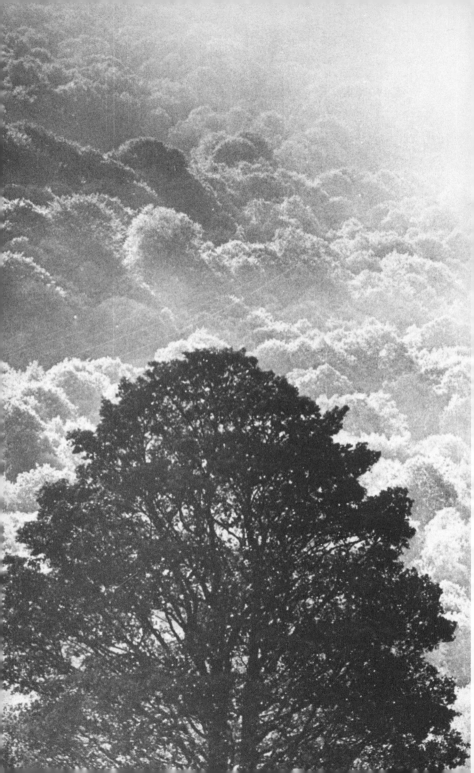

She is a woman of about thirty-seven. There is just still
about her the air of a schoolgirl: one of the less
bright girls who is physically more developed than the
others but whose physical maturity has already
made her slow and maternal rather than shifting and
sexy. There is just the last trace of this air about
her. In two years it will have vanished. She looks after
her mother and it is now for the mother rather than
the daughter that the doctor usually visits the cottage.

He first saw the daughter ten years ago. She had a
cold and cough and complained that she felt
weak. Her chest X-ray was normal. He had the im-
pression that she wanted to talk about something. She
would never look at him directly but kept casting
him quick anxious glances as though somehow
by these to bring him closer. He questioned her but
could not gain her confidence.

A few months later she was suffering from insomnia
and then asthma. All the tests for allergy proved
negative. The asthma got worse. Now when he saw her,
she smiled at him through her illness. Her eyes were
round like a rabbit's. She was timid of anything
outside the cage of her illness. If anybody approached
too near her eyes twitched like the skin round a
rabbit's nose. But her face was quite unlined. He was
convinced that her condition was the result of extreme
emotional stress. Both she and her mother insisted,
however, that she had no worries.

Two years later he discovered the explanation by
chance. He was out on a maternity case in the middle of
the night. There were three women neighbours in
attendance. Whilst waiting he had a cup of tea with
them in the kitchen. One of them worked in a
large mechanized dairy in the nearest railway town.
The girl with asthma had once worked there too. And
it turned out that the manager – who was in the
Salvation Army – had had an affair with her. Evidently
he had promised to marry her. Then he was overcome by remorse and religious scruples and had

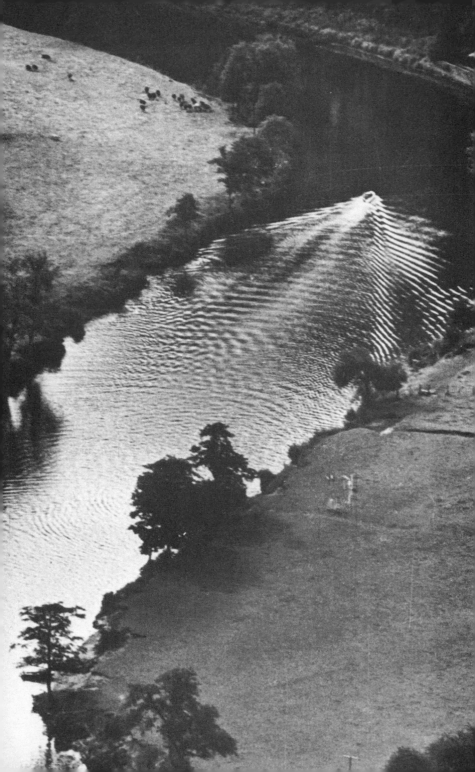

abandoned her. Was it even an affair – or did he only once, one evening, lead her by the hand out of the creamery up to his leather-chaired office?

The doctor once again questioned the girl's mother. Had her daughter been happy when she worked at that dairy? Yes, perfectly. He asked the girl if she had been happy there. She smiled in her cage and nodded her head. Then he asked her outright if the manager had ever made a pass at her. She froze – like an animal who realizes that it is impossible to bolt. Her hands stopped moving. Her head remained averted. Her breathing became inaudible. She never answered him.

Her asthma continued and caused structural deterioration of the lungs. She now survives on steroids. Her face is moon-shaped. The expression of her large eyes is placid. But her brows and eyelids and the skin pulled tight over her cheekbones twitch at every movement and sound which might constitute a warning of the unexpected. She looks after her mother, but very seldom leaves the cottage. When she sees the doctor, she smiles at him as now she would probably smile at the soldier of the Salvation Army.

Before, the water was deep. Then the torrent of God and the man. And afterwards the shallows, clear but constantly disturbed, endlessly irritated by their very shallowness as though by an allergy. There is a bend in the river which often reminds the doctor of his failure.   ∂

English autumn mornings are often like mornings nowhere else in the world.

The air is cold.

The floorboards are cold.

It is perhaps this coldness which sharpens the tang of the hot cup of tea. Outside, steps on the gravel crunch a little more loudly than a month ago because of the very slight frost. There is a smell of toast. And on the block of butter small grains of toast from the last impatient knife. Outside, there is sunlight which is simultaneously soft and very precise. Every leaf of each tree seems separate.

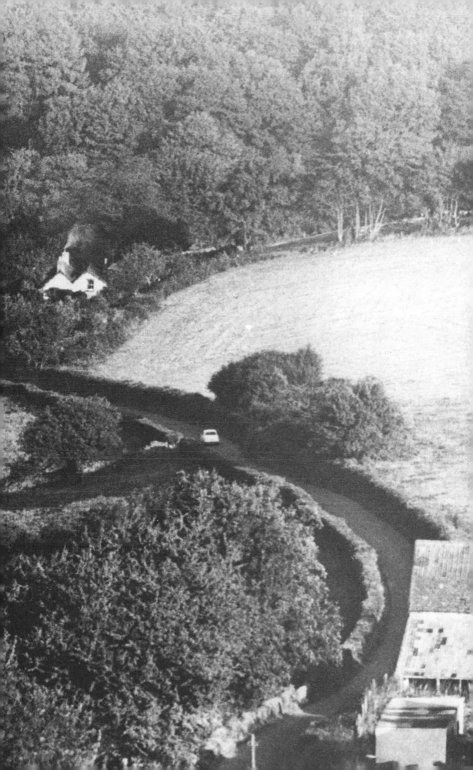

She lay in a four-poster bed: her face was ashen-coloured and her cheeks fallen in. Her eyes were tight shut in pain. She wheezed as she breathed, especially when breathing out.

The doctor stood looking and then asked for a cupful of warm water and cotton wool. As he injected morphia into her upper arm, she flinched a little. Strange that suffering so much pain in her chest she should flinch at the pin-prick. With the warm water and cotton wool he cleaned away the little droplet of blood from her worn, large arm, the colour of stone or bread, as though it had acquired the colour through its scrubbing and baking.

Then, using the same much-worked arm, he took her blood pressure. It was very low. She kept her eyes shut as if the light, so soft and so precise, was pressing between them. She had still said nothing.

He prepared a syringe for another injection. The fifty-year-old daughter was standing at the foot of the bed, waiting to be told what to do.

He inserted the needle into a vein near the wrist. This time she didn't flinch. After half the injection he paused, holding the syringe in the loose fold of skin as if it were the skin's feather, and with his other hand he felt her neck to check the strength of her pulse in the artery and the degree of congestion in the jugular vein. He then completed the injection.

The old woman opened her eyes. 'It's not your fault,' she said very distinctly, almost crisply.

He listened to her chest. Her overworked brown arms, her deeply lined face, her creased strained neck were suddenly denied by the soft whiteness of her breast. The grey-haired son down in the yard with the cows, the daughter at the foot of the bed in carpet slippers and with swollen ankles, had both once clambered and fed here, and yet the soft whiteness of her breast was like a young girl's. This she had preserved.

Downstairs in the parlour the doctor explained
the medicines he was leaving. The old woman's
wheezing was still audible through the floorboards.
Three dogs lay on the carpet, heads on out-
stretched paws, eyes open. They scarcely stirred when
the old man came in.

He seemed dazed and sleepy. The doctor asked him
how he was. 'Not so bad,' he said, 'except for the
screws.'

Neither father nor daughter nor the son outside asked
the doctor about the old woman. The doctor said
he would be coming back that evening.

When he came back the parlour was in darkness. This
disturbed him somewhat. He called out and receiving
no answer felt his way up the stairs. The stairs led
straight into the first bedroom. Across it he could see
the light under the door of the second room.

The room smelt now of sickness: under the dressing-
table on which stood all the family wedding photographs in leather frames and a nineteenth-century
child's mug with the Death and Burial of Cock Robin
engraved upon it, there was an enamel bowl with
urine in it, and spit stained a little with blood.
The daughter explained that every time her mother
coughed she peed a little involuntarily. The old
woman was paler and a piece of damp rag was laid over
her forehead. The room smouldered around her, all
its comfort burnt and drenched and then burnt again.

The doctor listened once more to her chest. She lay
back exhausted. 'I am sorry,' she said, not as
though it were an apology but simply a fact. He took
her temperature and blood pressure. 'I know,' he
said, 'but you'll sleep soon and feel rested.'

Her husband was sitting in the dark in the next room.
The doctor had walked through it without noticing
him, when he had come up the stairs. Now the
daughter shepherded both men down, but still without
putting a light on. For a moment it seemed that the

stairs and the parlour were part of the out-
buildings, unlit, unheated, belonging to the animals now
stabled for the night. It seemed that the home was
reduced to the four-poster bed in the lighted
room above, where the old woman, the soft whiteness
of whose breast had never changed, was dying.

When the daughter suddenly switched the light on,
the doctor and the old man were dazzled. For each
of them it was like finding himself on a stage.
The familiar furniture was part of a stage set and both
had to play roles which were utterly strange to what
they thought of as their true nature. Both would have
grasped any chance of reverting to the normal truth.

The old man sat down with an overcoat across his
knees. 'She has pneumonia now,' the doctor said, 'and
she must take another medicine beside the ones I
gave you this morning. Do you think she can swallow
these pills? They are rather large. Or would she
prefer to take it in liquid form? The liquid is made up
for children but we can increase the dose. Which do
you think would be best?'

The daughter, submissive and finding her only slight
hope in trust, said: 'It's up to you doctor.'

'No it's not,' he said. 'I'm asking you. Can she or can
she not swallow these pills?'

'Perhaps the liquid then,' said the daughter, abandoning her small hope. The doctor also gave her some
sleeping pills – for her father as well as her
mother. They would at least sleep tonight under the
same drug.

The old man, whilst the doctor was explaining the
medicines to the daughter, sat looking in front of
him, his hands clutching and unclutching the
heavy material of the overcoat across his knees.

When the doctor had finished his explanations, there
was a silence. Neither father nor daughter moved
to show him out or ask when he would be coming
again. They simply waited. The doctor said, 'The imme-
diate danger is past – another half hour and she

might have died this morning, now she's got to pay
the price of surviving the attack.'

'It sounds a funny mixture,' said the old man without
looking up, 'heart trouble and then pneumonia. A
funny mixture. She was quite well yesterday.'
He began to cry, very quietly, like a woman can: the
tears welling up in his eyes.

The doctor, who had already picked up one of his
bags, put it down again and leant back in the chair. 'Can
you make us a cup of tea?' he said

While the daughter was making the tea the two men
spoke about the orchard at the back and this year's
apples. When the daughter was there, they spoke about
the father's rheumatism. After the tea the doctor went.

The next morning was another autumn morning like
the preceding. Every leaf of each tree seemed
separate. The sunshine, filtered through a tree in the
orchard, played on the floor of the old woman's
bedroom. She clambered out of bed and suffered a
second attack. The doctor arrived within a quarter of an
hour. Her lips were purple, her face clay-coloured.
She died quickly, her hands very still.

In the parlour the old man rocked on his feet. The
doctor deliberately did not put out a hand to steady him.
Instead he faced him. The older man was the taller
by nine inches. The doctor said quietly, his eyes extra
wide behind his spectacles, 'It would have been
worse for her if she'd lived. It would have been worse.'

He might have said that there have been kings and
presidents of republics who have never recovered
from the death of their wives. He might have said that
death is the condition of life. He might have said
that man is indivisible and that, in his own view, this
was the only sense in which death could have no
dominion.

But whatever he said at that moment, the old man
would have continued to rock on his feet, until
the daughter lowered him into his chair in front of
the unlit fire.   Ꙩ

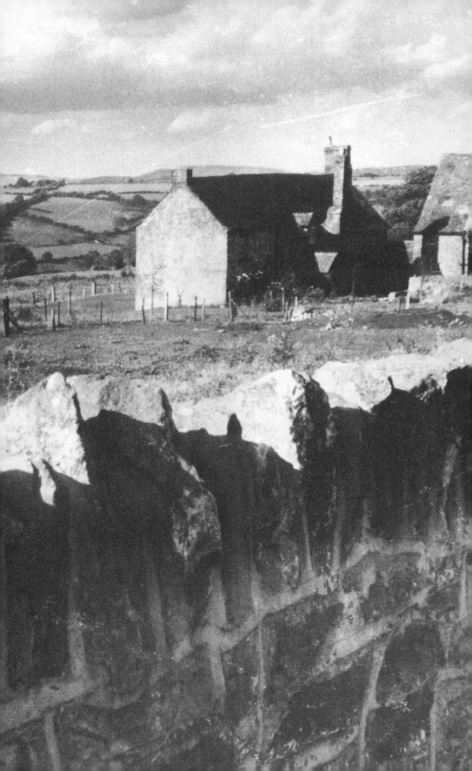

Only her feet betray her. There is something about the way she walks on her feet – a kind of irresponsibility towards them – which is still quite childish. Her figure is 36–25–36.

She was crying when she came into the surgery.

'What's wrong Duckie?'

'I just feel sort of miserable.'

She sat like other girls had sat there crying because they thought they were pregnant. To make it easier for her, the doctor slipped the question between several others.

'What's getting you down?'

No answer.

'Sore throat?'

'Not now.'

'Water-works all right?'

She nodded.

'Have you got a temperature?'

She shook her head.

'Periods regular?'

'Yeah.'

'When was your last one?'

'Last week.'

The doctor paused.

'Do you remember that rash you used to get on your tum? Has it ever come back?'

'No.'

He leant forward in his chair towards her.

'You just feel weepy?'

She inclined her head farther towards her own consoling bosom.

'Did Mum and Dad put you up to come to me?'

'No, I came myself.'

'Even having your hair dyed didn't make you feel better?'

She laughed a little because he had noticed. 'It did for a while.'

The doctor took her temperature, looked at her throat and told her to stay in bed for two days. Then he resumed the conversation.

'Do you like working in that laundry?'

'It's a job.'

'What about the other girls there?'

'I don't know.'

'Do you get on with them?'

'You get stopped if they find you talking.'

'Have you thought of doing anything else?'

'What can I do?'

'What would you like to do?'

'I'd like to do secretarial work.'

'Who would you like to be secretary to?'

She laughed and shook her head.

Her face was grubby with tear stains. But around her eyes and in the muzzle of her face which terminates in her full lip-sticked lips there is evidence of the same force that has filled out her bust and her hips.
She is nubile in everything except her education and her chances.

'When you're a bit better I'll keep you off work for a few days, if you like, and you can go to the Labour Exchange and find out how you can get trained. There are all kinds of training schemes.'

'Are there?' she said moonily.

'How did you do at school?'

'I wasn't any good.'

'Did you take O-levels?'

'No. I left.'

'But you weren't stupid were you?' He asked this as though if she admitted that she was, it would somehow reflect badly on him.

'No, not stupid.'

'Well,' he said.

'It's terrible that laundry. I hate it.'

'It's no good being sorry for yourself. If I give you a week off, will you really use it?'

She nodded, chewing her damp handkerchief.

'You can come up again on Wednesday and I'll phone the Labour Exchange and we'll talk about what they say.'

'I'm sorry,' she said, beginning to cry again.

'Don't be sorry. The fact that you're crying means you've got imagination. If you didn't have imagination, you wouldn't feel so bad. Now go to bed and stay there tomorrow.'

Through the surgery window he saw her walking up the lane to the common, to the house in which he had delivered her sixteen years ago. After she had turned the corner, he continued to stare at the stone walls on either side of the lane. Once they were dry walls. Now their stones were cemented together. Ɵ

He had heard rumours about them. That they were on
the run. That she was a prostitute from London.
That the Council would have to act to turn them out of
the abandoned cottage which the owner, a farmer,
had given them permission to use (some said because he
had met the girl in London) but in which they
were living like squatters.

Three children were playing by the back door with
some chicken wire. The mother was in the kitchen. She
was a woman in her late twenties with long black
hair, thin long hands and grey eyes that were both bright
and very liquid. Her skin had an unwashed look
which is more to do with anaemia than dirt.

'You won't be able to stay here in the winter,' he said.

'Jack says he's going to patch it up when he gets
the time.'

'It needs more than patching up.'

There was a table in the kitchen and two chairs.
By the stone sink there was an orange-box cupboard
with some cups and plates and packets in it. Half
the window above the sink was broken and there was
a piece of cardboard across it. The sunshine
streamed through the other half and the grey dust
slowly rose and fell through the beam, so slowly
that it seemed to be part of another uninhabited world.

Later in the front room she sat down on the bed
and allowed herself to ask the question for which she
had really sent for him.

'Doctor, can a woman of my age have heart
trouble?'

'It's possible. Did you ever have rheumatic fever
when you were a child?'

'I don't think so. But I get so out of breath. And if
I bend down to pick something up, I can scarcely
stand up proper again.'

'Let me have a listen. Just pull up your blouse.'

She wore a very worn black lace petticoat. The room
was as little furnished as the kitchen. There was a
large bed in one corner with some blankets on it and
some more blankets on the floor. There was also
a chest of drawers with a clock on it and a transistor
radio. The windows were overgrown with thick
ivy and since there was no plaster ceiling and holes in
the rafters, the room scarcely seemed geometric
and was more like a hide in a wood.

'We'll examine you properly when you come up to
the surgery but I can promise you now that you haven't
got a serious heart disease.'

'Oh I'm so relieved.'

'You can't go on like this. You know that don't you?
We've got to get you out of here –'

'There's lots more unfortunate than us,' she said.

The doctor laughed, and then so did she. She was still
young enough for her face to change totally with
her expression. Her face looked capable of
surprise again.

'If I won the football pools,' she said, 'I'd buy a big
house and start a big home for children, but they
say they make all kinds of difficulties these days for that
kind of thing.'

'Where were you living before you came here?'

'In Cornwall. It was lovely there by the sea. Look.'

She opened the top drawer of the chest and from
among her own stockings and children's socks she took
out a photograph. It showed herself in high-heeled
shoes, a tight skirt and a chiffon scarf round her head
with a man and a small child walking along a
beach.

'That's your husband?'

'No, that's not Jack, that's Cliff and Stephen.'

The doctor nodded, surprised.

'I'll say that for Jack,' she continued, 'he never makes no distinction between the kids that are his and those that are mine like. We share fifty-fifty. He's better to Steve than his own father. It's just that he can't touch me.'

She looked at the photograph, holding it out at arm's length.

The doctor asked whether she and her husband wanted to stay in the area and what would they think if he tried to get them a Council house. She answered without glancing away from the photo.

'You have to ask Jack about that. We do everything fifty-fifty.'

Still holding the photograph she let her arm fall on to her lap and looked at the doctor, her eyes now angry.

'Can you tell me if I'm too old? Jack says I'm too old. I only want it every two or three months.'

'That's all to do with your being tired and feeling you can't cope.'

'I've had a bellyful all right. Sometimes I think I just can't go on. I just want to lie down and stop.'

She got up and put the photograph back in the drawer. 'Do you like music?' she said and switched the radio on. Then after a few bars, she switched it off. She stood there against the chest, a quite different expression on her face: as though switching the radio on and off had reminded her of something.

'It just doesn't mean anything to me. It doesn't touch me. When he makes love to me it's like a wet rag across my face. I know what real love is like you see. With the father of Stephen, when I got Stephen it was beautiful. We came together and I was able to come to him with all of me. I know what they mean when they say it is the most wonderful thing in the world, it was like that when I got Stephen because I could come to him and he wanted me like that. And I shall never forget it – I lie awake and think of it yet – because it has never been like that again when it was like heaven when I got Stephen.'   Ə

37

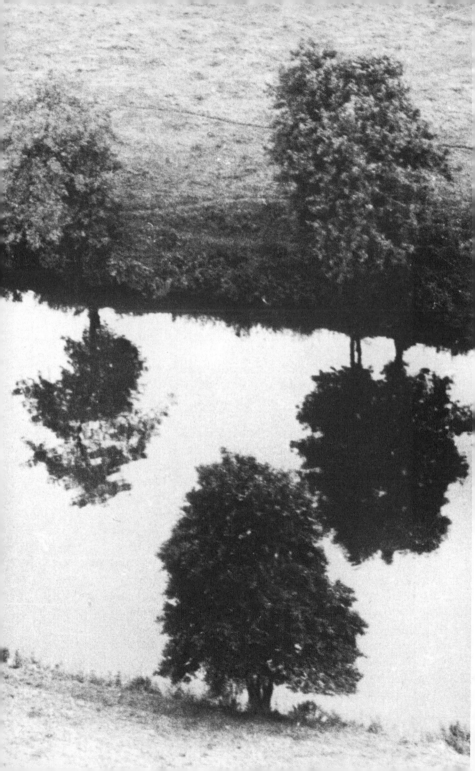

We fell in love with it ten years ago – for the view.
And I must say we've never regretted it, not even in the
winter. It's so peaceful. Do you know last spring
when I was walking along the path from the village
I saw something standing in the front gate. I could
see it as I turned the corner by the wood. It looked like
a dog but it didn't, if you know what I mean. And
do you know what it was? It was a badger. It just stood
there between the gate-posts and stared at me. I
didn't know what to do. Can they be dangerous? I just
didn't know. Hugh was playing golf and so I went
to ask Mr Hornby, and he came back with me, but by
that time it had gone. But that isn't the end of the
story. The badger has come to stay I think. He's invited
himself. You remember the deep snow we had last
winter, I don't know what we'd have done then without
Mr Hornby, he cleared the path through the wood,
otherwise you just couldn't get through, it was up to my
waist, and it was very cold too, the cold was cruel,
anyway as I was saying in the night I used to
hear something on the roof, something moving about,

I woke up Hugh several times and he said it was
the snow shifting but I knew it wasn't because it was
too cold you see for the snow to be moving, and
in the morning I went to look and do you know there
were his footsteps in the snow on the roof, would
you believe it? I suppose he was so cold up there in the
wood behind that he came down in the dark for
a bit of warmth. He could have nestled up against the
chimney – Hugh says not, but I'm sure he could
– and got nice and warm. I often think of him up there
when I'm sitting by the fire thinking. Of course
it's silly but you can see what I mean about it being very
peaceful, can't you? I mean you wouldn't get badgers
in Birmingham where we used to live when Hugh
was still at work . . .' she continues endlessly.

When she phones it is usually about him rather than
herself.

'I'm worried about him, doctor, he's got a pain in his
back and I think it might be a slipped disk. It
all came on in that wet spell last week when he insisted
upon digging the vegetable garden, the first
chance for two months, he said, and now he can't
straighten up.'

Sometimes it sounds more serious.

'He's been in bed for three days and he has great
difficulty in breathing. When he breathes at night – and I
simply can't get to sleep listening to him – I keep
on thinking he's talking, his breathing sounds like
words, doctor.'

She is there at the door waiting.

'I'm so glad you've come. His whole body is col-
lapsing. I better let you talk to him yourself, because he
won't tell me what he's complaining of, he won't
come out with it, he's funny like that you know, he just
says all his organs are going. Which? I say. What
do you mean? But he won't tell me, he just says all his
organs.'

The husband, aged seventy-three, explains that he
can't hold his water and that he has some pain

40

in the lower part of the abdomen. The doctor checks his
chest and stomach. He does a rectal examination to
feel the prostate and to discover whether any growth is
pressing on the bladder. He tests the urine for
sugar and albumen. The sugar is just problematic. He
diagnoses a mild urinary infection.

Thirty-six hours later she phones.

'He just can't take any liquid at all now. He can't
drink. He hasn't taken a drop since yesterday breakfast.
And he keeps on falling asleep. Right in the middle
of my talking to him he just falls off – I don't
know what to do. He just can't keep awake, not even
when I'm talking to him, he just falls asleep and
then he's sleepy and he falls asleep again even when
I'm talking to him.'

The doctor smiles into the phone. Yet, just
conceivably, if almost impossibly, the sleeping might be
the beginning of a diabetic coma: the diabetes made
manifest by the urinary infection. To be certain he must
do another blood test for sugar.

At that gate where the badger stood, he pauses and
looks down at the view with which they fell
in love, and then he remembers her saying in a more
intense, more sibilant voice than her ordinary one:

'All we've got is each other. So we have to be very
strict. We watch over each other carefully when
we are ill, we do.'

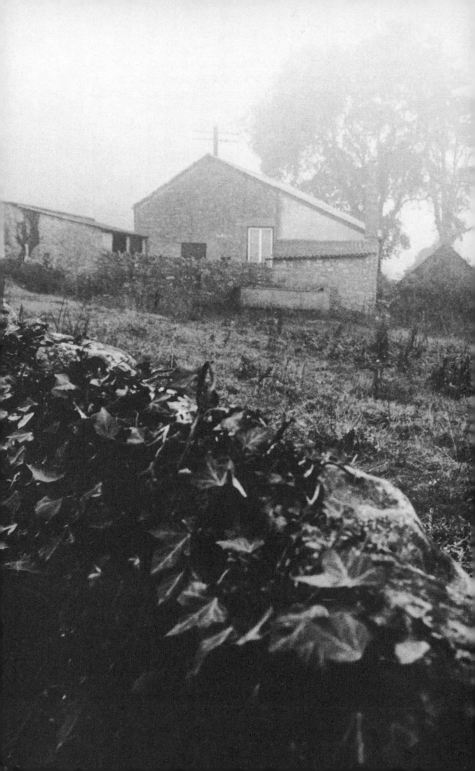

It is apart from the house: a building the size of two garages. It consists of a waiting-room, two consulting rooms and a dispensary. It is on the side of the hill which overlooks the river and the large wooded valley. From the other side of the valley it is almost too small to be visible.

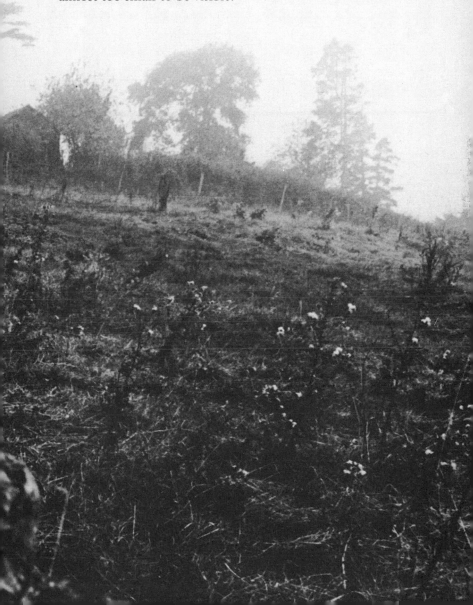

On the door of the building is a notice which reads:
Dr John Sassall M.B., Ch.B., D.Obst.R.C.O.G.

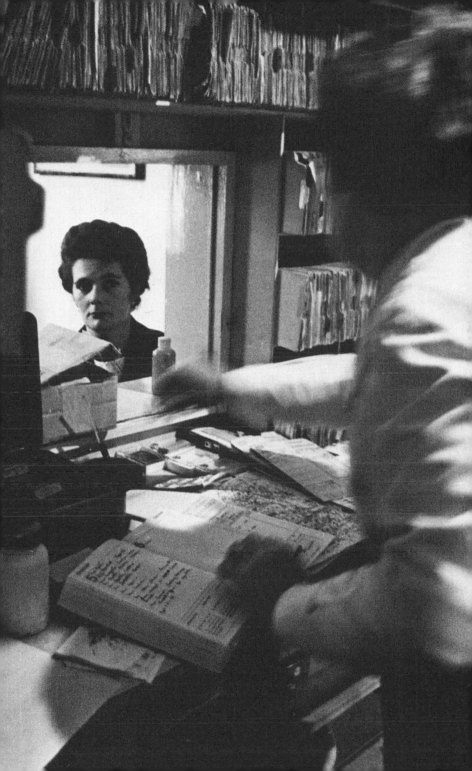

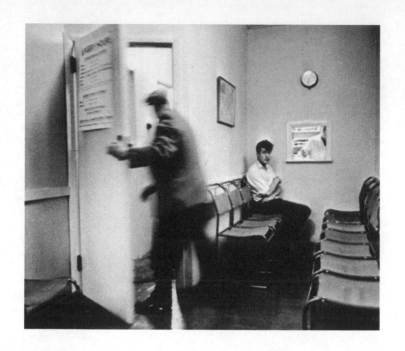

The consulting rooms do not seem clinical. They seem lived-in and cosy. But they are neater than most living-rooms and, despite their smallness, there is more clear space. This is the working area where the patient is examined or treated or manipulated.

The rooms remind one of a ship's officer's cabin. There is the same cosiness, the same ingenuity in fitting many things into a small space, the same odd juxta-position of domestic furniture and personal effects with instruments and appliances.

All this makes the examining couch look like a bunk. It has two sheets on it and an electric blanket. Whenever patients are due, Sassall switches the blanket on a quarter of an hour beforehand, so that if a patient has to strip and be examined, it will not strike as cold. He has a fastidious sense for detail. He is a short man; the chair in which the patients sit is exactly six inches lower than his own chair by the desk. Before he gives an injection he says: 'You'll just feel a tap.' As his hand comes down, holding the syringe, he opens his little finger and with the side of his hand flicks hard against the skin by the side of where the needle will go in a fraction of a second later, and this distracts the patient from registering the prick of the needle.

The surgery is unusually well equipped. There is stoving equipment for sterilizing and the instruments necessary for the suture of tendons, minor amputations, the removal of cysts, cauterization of the cervix, the application and removal of plaster for minor fractures. There is an anaesthetic machine: an osteopathic table: a sigmoidoscope. He says that he is constantly frustrated because he has not got his own X-ray plant or his own equipment for elementary bacteriology.

If possible, he always wants to prove everything for himself.

Once he was putting a syringe deep into a man's chest: there was little question of pain but it made the

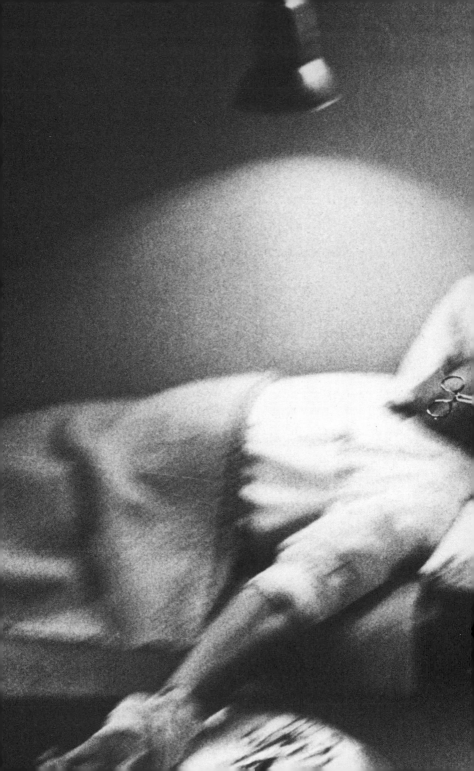

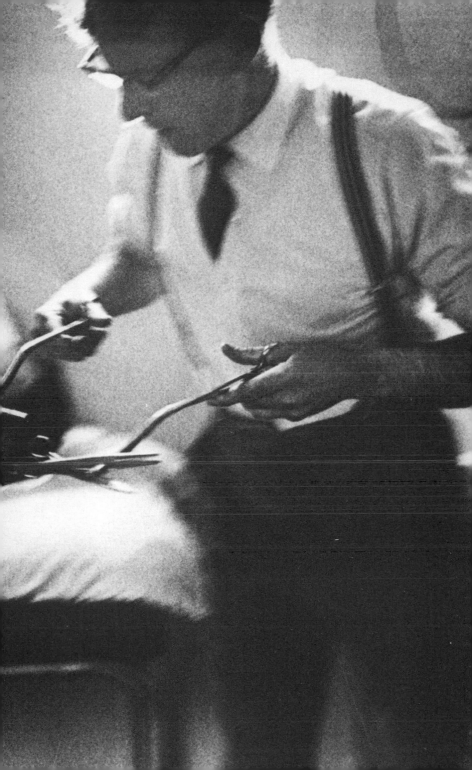

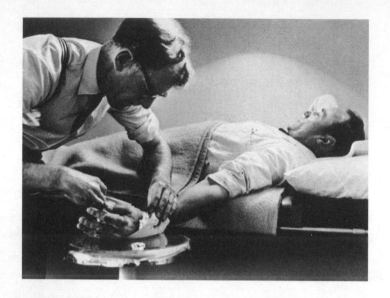

man feel bad: the man tried to explain his revulsion: 'That's where I live, where you're putting that
needle in.' 'I know,' Sassall said, 'I know what
it feels like. I can't bear anything done near my eyes, I
can't bear to be touched there. I think that's where
I live, just under and behind my eyes.'   ⋻

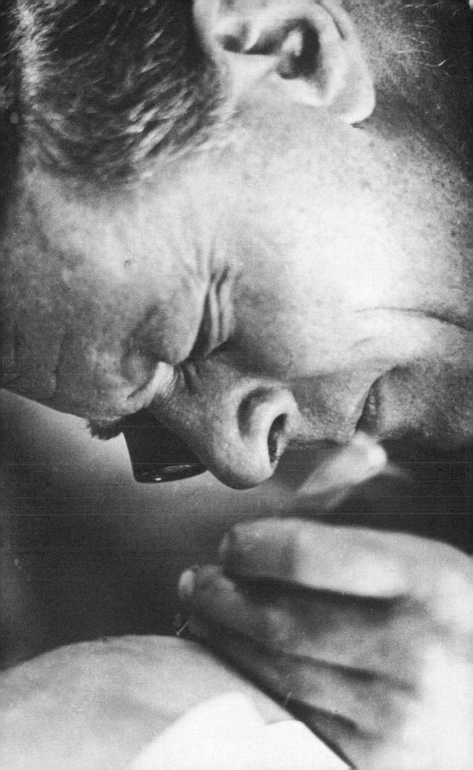

As a boy Sassall was much influenced by the books of
Conrad. Against the boredom and complacency
of middle-class life ashore in England, Conrad offered
the 'unimaginable' whose instrument was the sea.
Yet in this offered poetry there was nothing unmanly or
effete: on the contrary, the only men who could
face the unimaginable were tough, controlled, taciturn
and outwardly ordinary. The quality which
Conrad constantly warns against is at the same time the
very quality to which he appeals: the quality of
imagination. It is almost as though the sea is the symbol
of this contradiction. It is to the imagination that
the sea appeals: but to face the sea in its unimaginable
fury, to meet its own challenge, imagination must
be abandoned, for it leads to self-isolation and fear.

What resolves the contradiction and, in resolving it,
places the whole drama on a level incomparably
higher and more noble than the average petty life of
self-seeking advancement, is the ideal of service.
This ideal has a double meaning. The Service stands for
all those traditional values which a privileged few
who have faced and met the challenge esteem: esteem
not as an abstract principle but as the very condition of practising their craft efficiently. And at the
same time service also stands for the responsibility which
the few must always carry for the many who
depend upon them – the passengers, the crew, the
traders, the ship-owners, the brokers.

Of course I simplify. And Conrad would not be the
great artist he is if this were a fair summary of
his attitude to the sea. But the simplification is enough
to allow us to see why Conrad might appeal to a
boy who was in revolt against his middle-class family
background but who had no interest in becoming a Bohemian. He admired physical prowess. He
enjoyed being practical and using his hands. He
was inquisitive about things rather than feelings. He was
stirred – like many boys of his class and generation –

by the ideal of a moral example which might
shame the opportunism of his elders.

In fact by the age of fifteen he had decided to become
a doctor rather than a sailor. His father was a
dentist and consequently he had the opportunity of
meeting doctors socially. When he was fourteen he was
already hanging round the dispensary of the local
doctor: nominally helping to wrap up medicine bottles,
actually trying to listen to the consultations taking
place in the next room. Yet a doctor can well
be imagined as the equivalent of a Master Mariner.

Sassall's image of a doctor at that time was:

'A man who was all-knowing but looking haggard.
Once a doctor came in the middle of the night
and I could see that he slept too – his pyjama trousers
were poking out through the bottom of his
trousers. But above all I remember he was in command
and composed – whereas everybody else was
fussing and agitated.'

Compare this to Conrad's first introduction of the
captain of the *Narcissus*:

Captain Allistoun, serious, and with an old red muffler
round his throat, all day long pervaded the poop. At night,
many times he rose out of the darkness of the companion,
such as a phantom above a grave, and stood watchful
and mute under the stars, his night-shirt fluttering like a flag
– then, without a sound, sank down again. . . . He, the
ruler of that minute world, seldom descended from the
Olympian heights of his poop. Below him – at his feet, so to
speak – common mortals led their busy and insignificant
lives.

In both impressions there is the same sense of
authority: an authority which pyjama trousers or a night-
shirt in no way diminish. Or consider Conrad's
description of one of the worst moments in *Typhoon*.
With the exception of the one word *gale*, it might
describe the crisis of an illness, with the voice of Captain
MacWhirr transformed into that of a doctor.

And again he heard that voice, forced and ringing feebly, but with a penetrating effect of quietness in the enormous discord of noises, as if sent out from some remote spot of peace beyond the black wastes of the gale; again he heard a man's voice – the frail and indomitable sound that can be made to carry an infinity of thought, resolution, and purpose, that shall be pronouncing confident words on the last day when heavens fall, and justice is done – again he heard it, and it was crying to him, as if from very, very far – 'All right'.

From such material Sassall constructed his ideal of responsibility.

During the war Sassall served in the Navy as a surgeon. 'That was the happiest time of my life, doing major surgery in the Dodecanese. I was dealing with very real distress and on the whole making a success of it.' In Rhodes he taught peasants elementary medicine. He saw himself as a life-saver. He had proved his skill to himself and his ability to take decisions. With this proof came the conviction that those who lived simply, those who were dependent upon him, possessed qualities and a secret of living which he lacked. Thus, whilst having authority over them, he could feel he was serving them.

After the war, he married* and chose a remote country practice under the National Health Service, becoming the junior partner of an old doctor who was much liked in the district but who hated the sight of blood and believed that the secret of medicine was faith. This gave the younger man plenty of opportunity to go on working as a life-saver.

He was always overworked and proud of it. Most of the time he was out on calls – often having to make his way over fields, or walk, carrying his black

* I do not attempt in this essay to discuss the role of Sassall's wife or his children. My concern is his professional life.

boxes of instruments and drugs, along forest
paths. In the winter he had to dig his way through the
snow. Along with his instruments he carried a
blow-lamp for thawing out pipes.

He was scarcely ever in the surgery. He imagined
himself as a sort of mobile one-man hospital.
He performed appendix and hernia operations on
kitchen tables. He delivered babies in caravans. It would
almost be true to say that he sought out accidents.

He had no patience with anything except emergencies
or serious illness. When a man continued to
complain but had no dangerous symptoms, he reminded
himself of the endurance of the Greek peasants and
the needs of those in 'very real distress', and
so recommended more exercise and, if possible, a cold
bath before breakfast. He dealt only with crises
in which he was the central character: or, to put it
another way, in which the patient was *simplified* by the
degree of his physical dependence on the doctor.
He was also simplified himself, because the chosen pace
of his life made it impossible and unnecessary for
him to examine his own motives.

After a few years he began to change. He was in his
mid thirties: at that time of life when, instead of
being spontaneously oneself as in one's twenties, it is
necessary, in order to remain honest, to confront
oneself and judge from a second position. Furthermore
he saw his patients changing. Emergencies always
present themselves as *faits accomplis*. At last, because he
was living among the same people all the time,
and because he was often called to the same cottage
several times for different emergencies, he began to notice
how people developed. A girl whom three years
before he had treated for measles got married and came
to him for her first confinement. A man who had
never been ill shot his brains out.

One day he was called to a couple of old-age
pensioners. They had lived in the Forest for thirty years.
Nobody had anything very special to say about

them. They went every year on the Old Folks' Annual
Outing. They usually went to the pub at about
eight every Saturday evening. A long time before, the
wife had worked as a maid in the big house of a
near-by village. The husband had worked on the railway.
The husband said that his wife 'was bleeding from
down below'.

Sassall talked to her a little and then asked her to
undress so that he could examine her. He went into the
kitchen to wait until she was ready. There the
husband looked at him anxiously and took the clock
from the mantelpiece to wind it. At this age if
the wife has to go into hospital, it can be the beginning
of the end for them both.

When he went back into the parlour, the wife was
lying on the ottoman. Her stockings were rolled
down and her dress up. 'She' was a man. He examined
her. The trouble was severe piles. Neither he nor
the husband nor she referred to the sexual organs which
should not have been there. They were ignored.
Or, rather, he was forced to accept them, as they had
done according to their own reasoning which
he would never know.

He became aware of the possibility of his patients
changing. They, as they became more used to
him, sometimes made confessions for which there was
no medical reference so far as he had learnt. He
began to take a different view of the meaning of the
term crisis.

He began to realize that the way Conrad's Master
Mariners came to terms with their imagination – denying
it any expression but projecting it all on to the sea
which they then faced as though it were simultaneously
their personal justification and their personal
enemy – was not suitable for a doctor in his position.
He had done just that – using illness and medical
dangers as they used the sea. He began to realize that he
must face his imagination, even explore it. It must
no longer lead always to the 'unimaginable', as it had

with the Master Mariners contemplating the
possible fury of the elements – or, as in his case, to his
contemplating only fights within the jaws of death
itself. (The clichés are essential to the vision.) He began
to realize that imagination had to be lived with
on every level: his own imagination first – because
otherwise this could distort his observation – and then
the imagination of his patients.

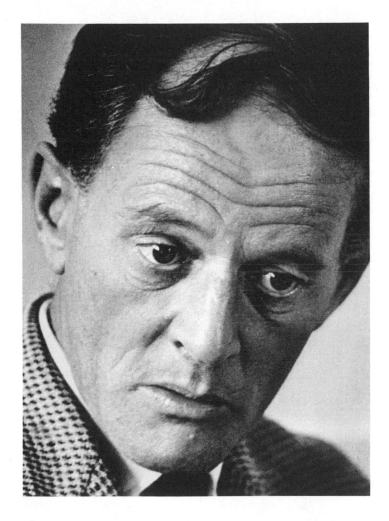

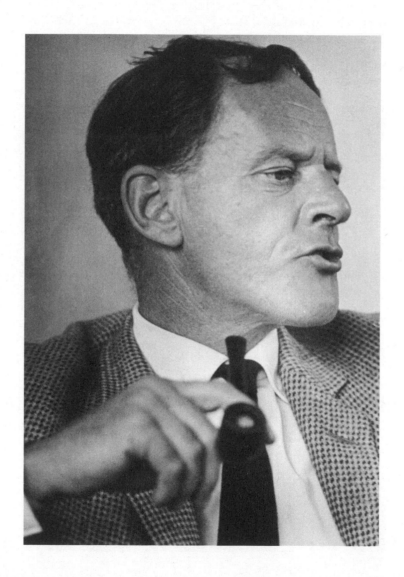

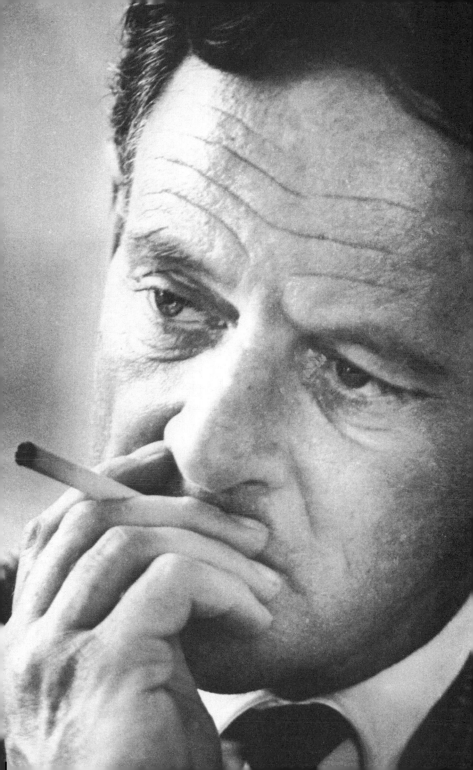

The older partner died. Sassall had to spend far more time in the surgery, listening. He also had to find another doctor to share his practice with. He decided to split the practice in two so that the other doctor should work with his own surgery in his own area. Then, still overworked, but with more time for the average patient, he began to observe himself and others.

He began to read – especially Freud. So far as a man can by himself, he analysed many of his own character traits and their roots in the past. It was a painful process – as Freud himself describes when discussing his own self-analysis. For six months or so, as a result of his resurrected memories, Sassall became sexually impotent. It is impossible to say now whether this period of crisis was induced by his decision to examine within himself the basis of what up to now he had projected outwards as 'the unimaginable', or whether he entered a period of crisis and therefore decided to look more closely at himself. Either way it bears some resemblance to the period of isolation

and crisis which precedes in Siberian and African
medicine the professional emergence of the *shaman* or the
inyanga. The Zulus have a name for this process.
The *inyanga*, they say, suffers because the spirits will give
him no peace and he becomes 'a house of dreams'.

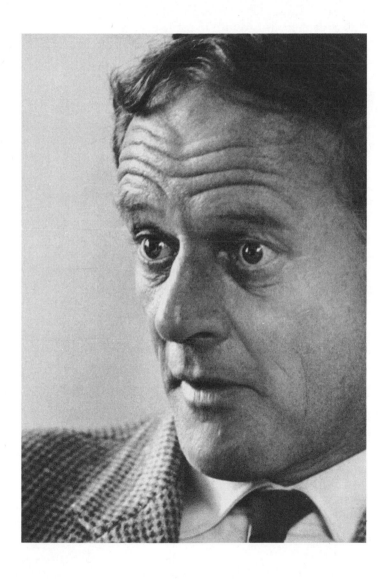

When Sassall emerged, he was still an extremist. He had exchanged an obvious and youthful form of extremism for a more complex and mature one: the life-and-death emergency for the intimation that the patient should be treated as a total personality, that illness is frequently a form of expression rather than a surrender to natural hazards.

This is dangerous ground, for it is easy to get lost among countless intangibles and to forget or neglect all the precise skills and information which have brought medicine to the point where there is the time and opportunity to pursue such intimations. The quack is either a charlatan or he is a healer who refuses to relate his own few insights to the general body of medical knowledge.

Sassall enjoyed this danger. Safe thinking was now like settling down ashore. 'Common-sense has been a dirty word with me for many years now – except perhaps when it is applied to very factual and easily assessed problems. When dealing with human beings it is my biggest enemy – and tempter. It tempts me to accept the obvious, the easiest, the most readily available answer. It has failed me on almost every occasion I have used it – and God knows how often I have fallen and still fall for the trap.'

Every week now he reads in considerable detail the three main medical journals, and from time to time goes on a refresher course at some hospital. He sees to it that he stays well-informed. But his satisfaction comes mostly from those cases where he faces forces which no previous explanation will exactly fit, because they depend upon the history of a patient's particular personality. He tries to keep that personality company in its loneliness.

He is acknowledged as a good doctor. The organization of his practice, the facilities he offers, his diagnostic and clinical skill are probably somewhat under-rated.

His patients may not realize how lucky they are. But in a sense this is inevitable. Only the most self-conscious consider it lucky to have their elementary needs met. And it is on a very basic, elementary level that he is judged a good doctor.

They would say that he was straight, not afraid of work, easy to talk to, not stand-offish, kind, understanding, a good listener, always willing to come out when needed, very thorough. They would also say that he was moody, difficult to understand when on one of his theoretical subjects like sex, capable of doing things just to shock, unusual.

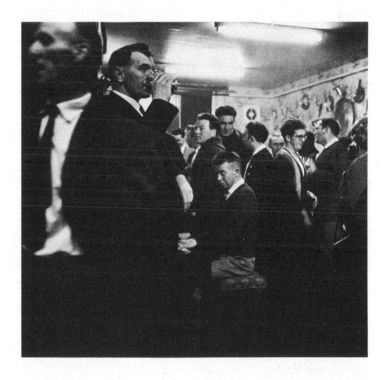

How he actually answers their needs as a doctor is
far more complicated than any of these epithets
imply. To understand this we must first consider the
special character and depth of any doctor-patient
relationship.

The primitive medicine-man, who was often also
priest, sorcerer and judge, was the first specialist to be
released from the obligation of procuring food for
the tribe. The magnitude of this privilege and
of the power which it gave him is a direct reflection of
the importance of the needs he served. An awareness
of illness is part of the price that man first paid
and still pays for his self-consciousness. This awareness
increases the pain or disability. But the self-consciousness
of which it is the result is a social phenomenon and
so with this self-consciousness arises the possibility of
treatment, of medicine.*

We cannot imaginatively reconstruct the subjective
attitude of a tribesman to his treatment. But within our
culture today what is our own attitude? How do
we acquire the necessary trust to submit ourselves to
the doctor?

We give the doctor access to our bodies. Apart from
the doctor, we only grant such access voluntarily
to lovers – and many are frightened to do even this.
Yet the doctor is a comparative stranger.

* For the philosophical implication of early medicine see
first two volumes of Henry Sigerist's *History of Medicine*:
vol. 1, *Primitive and Archaic Medicine* (New York:
O.U.P., 1951); vol. 2, *Early Greek, Hindu, and Persian
Medicine* (New York: O.U.P., 1961).

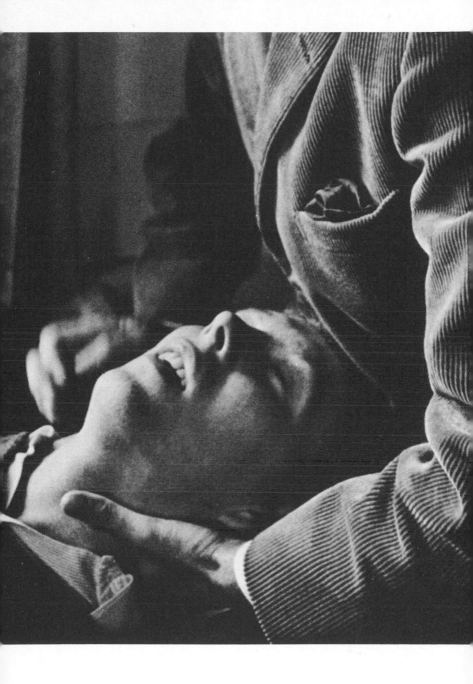

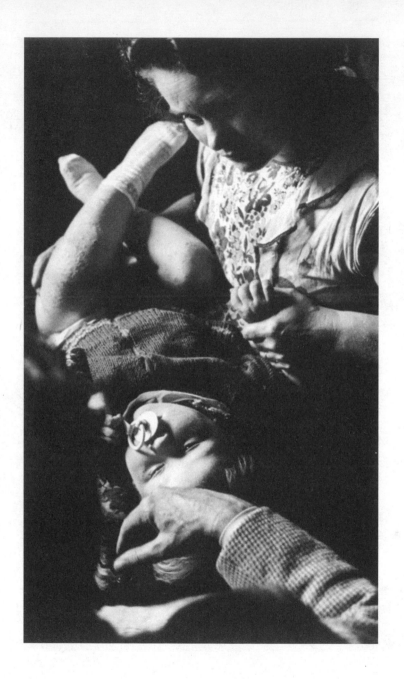

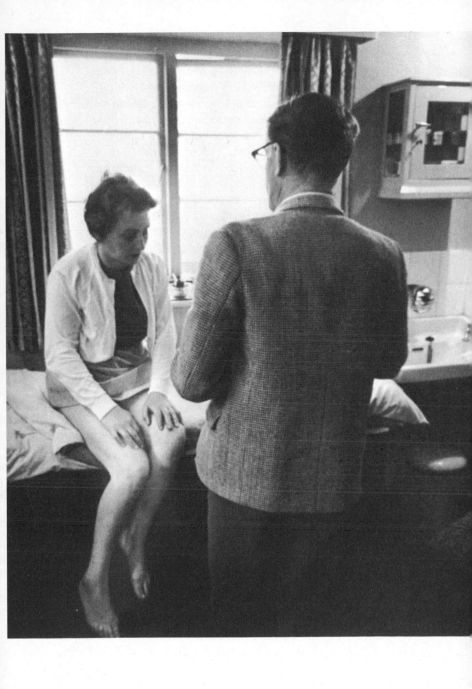

The degree of intimacy implied by the relationship is emphasized by the concern of all medical ethics (not only ours) to make an absolute distinction between the roles of doctor and lover. It is usually assumed that this is because the doctor can see women naked and can touch them where he likes and that this may sorely tempt him to make love to them. It is a crude assumption, lacking imagination. The conditions under which a doctor is likely to examine his patients are always sexually discouraging.

The emphasis in medical ethics on sexual correctness is not so much to restrict the doctor as to offer a promise to the patient: a promise which is far more than a reassurance that he or she will not be taken advantage of. It is a positive promise of physical intimacy without a sexual basis. Yet what can such intimacy mean? Surely it belongs to the experiences of childhood. We submit to the doctor by quoting to ourselves a state of childhood and simultaneously extending our sense of family to include him. We imagine him as an honorary member of the family.

In cases where the patient is fixated on a parent, the doctor may become a substitute for this parent. But in such a relationship the high degree of sexual content creates difficulties. In illness we ideally imagine the doctor as an elder brother or sister.

Something similar happens at death. The doctor is the familiar of death. When we call for a doctor, we are asking him to cure us and to relieve our suffering, but, if he cannot cure us, we are also asking him to witness our dying. The value of the witness is that he has seen so many others die. (This, rather than the prayers and last rites, was also the real value which the priest once had.) He is the living intermediary between us and the multitudinous dead. He belongs to us and he has belonged to them. And the hard but real comfort which they offer through him is still that of fraternity.

It would be a great mistake to 'normalize' what I have just said by concluding that quite naturally the patient wants a *friendly* doctor. His hopes and demands, however contradicted by previous experience, however protected they may be by scepticism, however undeclared even to himself, are much more profound and precise.

In illness many connexions are severed. Illness separates and encourages a distorted, fragmentated form of self-consciousness. The doctor, through his relationship with the invalid and by means of the special intimacy he is allowed, has to compensate for these broken connections and reaffirm the social content of the invalid's aggravated self-consciousness.

When I speak of a fraternal relationship – or rather of the patient's deep, unformulated expectation of fraternity – I do not of course mean that the doctor can or should behave like an actual brother. What is required of him is that he should recognize his patient with the certainty of an ideal brother. The function of fraternity is recognition.

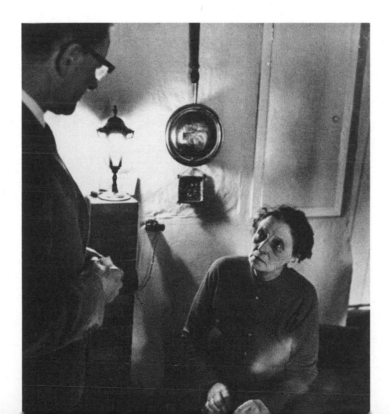

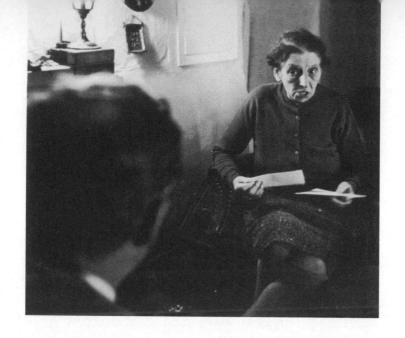

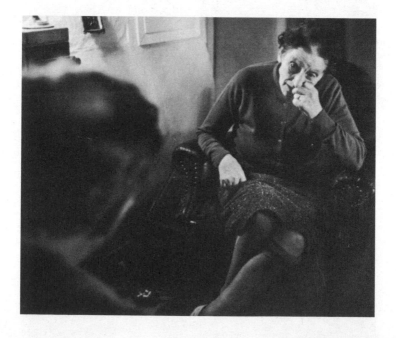

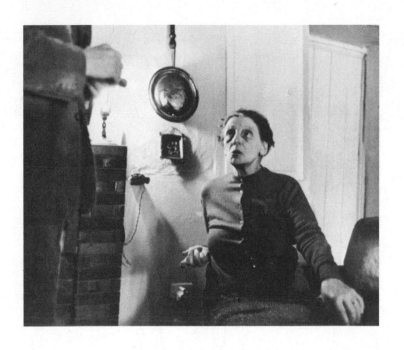

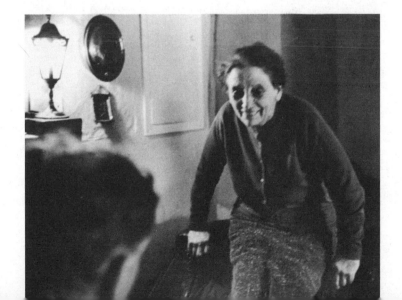

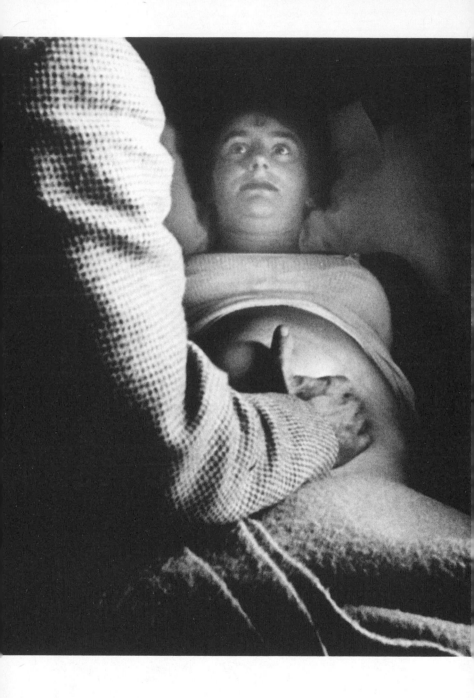

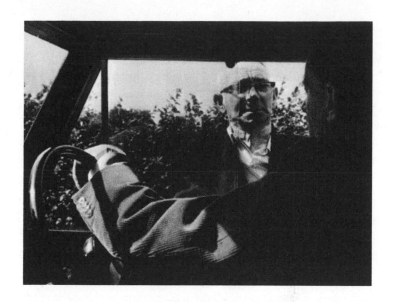

This individual and closely intimate recognition
is required on both a physical and psychological level.
On the former it constitutes the art of diagnosis.
Good general diagnosticians are rare, not because most
doctors lack medical knowledge, but because
most are incapable of taking in all the possibly
relevant facts – emotional, historical, environmental as
well as physical. They are searching for specific
conditions instead of the truth about a man which may
then suggest various conditions. It may be that
computers will soon diagnose better than doctors. But
the facts fed to the computers will still have to be the
result of intimate, individual recognition of the patient.

On the psychological level recognition means support.
As soon as we are ill we fear that our illness is
unique. We argue with ourselves and rationalize, but
a ghost of the fear remains. And it remains for a
very good reason. The illness, as an undefined force, is
a potential threat to our very being and we are
bound to be highly conscious of the uniqueness of that
being. The illness, in other words, shares in our

own uniqueness. By fearing its threat, we embrace it and make it specially our own. That is why patients are inordinately relieved when doctors give their complaint a name. The name may mean very little to them; they may understand nothing of what it signifies; but because it has a name, it has an independent existence from them. They can now struggle or complain *against* it. To have a complaint recognized, that is to say defined, limited and depersonalized, is to be made stronger.

The whole process, as it includes doctor and patient, is a dialectical one. The doctor in order to recognize the illness fully – I say fully because the recognition must be such as to indicate the specific treatment – must first recognize the patient as a person: but for the patient – provided that he trusts the doctor and that trust finally depends upon the efficacy of his treatment – the doctor's recognition of his illness is a help because it separates and depersonalizes that illness.*

So far we have discussed the problem at its simplest, assuming that illness is something which befalls the patient. We have ignored the role of unhappiness in illness, the factors of emotional or mental disturbance. Estimates among G.P.s of how many of their cases actually depend on such factors vary from five to thirty per cent: this is perhaps because there is no quick way of distinguishing between cause and effect and because in nearly *all* cases there is emotional stress present of one kind or another which has to be dealt with.

Most unhappiness is like illness in that it too exacerbates a sense of uniqueness. All frustration magnifies its own dissimilarity and so nourishes itself. Objectively speaking this is illogical since in our

* For a full study of the subject see Michael Balint's brilliant book *The Doctor, His Patient and The Illness* (London: Pitman, 1964).

society frustration is far more usual than satisfaction, unhappiness far more common than contentment. But it is not a question of objective comparison. It is a question of failing to find any confirmation of oneself in the outside world. The lack of confirmation leads to a sense of futility. And this sense of futility is the essence of loneliness: for, despite the horrors of history, the existence of other men always promises the possibility of purpose. Any example offers hope. But the conviction of being unique destroys all examples.

An unhappy patient comes to a doctor to offer him an illness in the hope that this part of him at least (the illness) may be recognizable. His proper self he believes to be unknowable. In the light of the world he is nobody: by his own lights the world is nothing. Clearly the task of the doctor – unless he merely accepts the illness on its face value and incidentally guarantees for himself a 'difficult' patient – is to recognize the man. If the man can begin to feel recognized – and such recognition may well include aspects of his character which he has not yet recognized himself – the hopeless nature of his unhappiness will have been changed: he may even have the chance of being happy.

I am fully aware that I am here using the word Recognition to cover whole complicated techniques of psychotherapy, but essentially these techniques are precisely means for furthering the process of recognition. How does a doctor begin to make an unhappy man feel recognized?

A straightforward frontal greeting will achieve little. The patient's name has become meaningless: it has become a wall to hide what is happening, uniquely, behind it. Nor can his unhappiness be named – as is the case with an illness. What can the word 'depressed' mean to the depressed? It is no more than the echo of the patient's own voice.

The recognition has to be oblique. The unhappy man expects to be treated as though he were a nonentity

with certain symptoms attached. The state of
being a nonentity then paradoxically and bitterly
confirms his uniqueness. It is necessary to break the
circle. This can be achieved by the doctor
presenting himself to the patient as a comparable man.
It demands from the doctor a true imaginative
effort and precise self-knowledge. The patient must be
given the chance to recognize, despite his
aggravated self-consciousness, aspects of himself in the
doctor, but in such a way that the doctor seems to
be Everyman. This chance is probably seldom the result
of a single exchange, and it may come about more
as the result of the general atmosphere than of any special
words said. As the confidence of the patient
increases, the process of recognition becomes more
subtle. At a later stage of treatment, it is the
doctor's acceptance of what the patient tells him and the
accuracy of his appreciation as he suggests how
different parts of his life may fit together, it is this which
then persuades the patient that he and the doctor
and other men are comparable because whatever he says
of himself or his fears or his fantasies seems to be
at least as familiar to the doctor as to him.
He is no longer an exception. He can be recognized.
And this is the prerequisite for cure or adaptation.

   We can now return to our original question. How is it
that Sassall is acknowledged as a good doctor? By
his cures? This would seem to be the answer.
But I doubt it. You have to be a startlingly bad doctor
and make many mistakes before the results tell
against you. In the eyes of the layman the results always
tend to favour the doctor. No, he is acknowledged
as a good doctor because he meets the deep
but unformulated expectation of the sick for a sense of
fraternity. He recognizes them. Sometimes he fails
– often because he has missed a critical opportunity and
the patient's suppressed resentment becomes too
hard to break through – but there is about
him the constant will of a man trying to recognize.

'The door opens,' he says, 'and sometimes I feel I'm
in the valley of death. It's all right when once
I'm working. I try to overcome this shyness because for
the patient the first contact is extremely important.
If he's put off and doesn't feel welcome, it may take a
long time to win his confidence back and perhaps never.
I try to give him a fully open greeting. All diffidence
in my position is a fault. A form of negligence.'

It is as though when he talks or listens to a patient, he
is also touching them with his hands so as to be
less likely to misunderstand: and it is as though, when
he is physically examining a patient, they were
also conversing.

Sassall needs to work in this way. He cures others to
cure himself. The phrase is usually no more than
a cliché: a conclusion. But now in one particular case
we can begin to understand the process.

Previously the sense of mastery which Sassall gained
was the result of the skill with which he dealt with
emergencies. The possible complications would all appear
to develop within his own field: they were medical
complications. He remained the central character.

Now the patient is the central character. He tries to
recognize each patient and, having recognized
him, he tries to set an example for him – not a morally
improving example, but an example wherein the
patient can recognize himself. One could simplify this –
for now we are not dealing with the complexities
of the average case but with Sassall's motives – by saying
that he 'becomes' each patient in order to
'improve' that patient. He 'becomes' the patient by
offering him his own example back. He 'improves' him
by curing or at least alleviating his suffering. Yet
patient succeeds patient whilst he remains the same
person, and so the effect is cumulative. His
sense of mastery is fed by the ideal of striving towards
the *universal*.

The ideal of the universal man has a long history. It was the working ideal of Greek democracy – even though it depended on slavery. It was revived in the Renaissance and became for a number of men a reality. It was one of the principles of the eighteenth-century Enlightenment and after the French Revolution was maintained, at least as a vision, by Goethe, Marx, Hegel. The enemy of the universal man is the division of labour. By the mid nineteenth century the division of labour in capitalist society had not only destroyed the possibility of a man having many roles: it denied him even one role, and condemned him instead to being part of a part of a mechanical process. Little wonder that Conrad believed that 'the true place of God begins at any spot a thousand miles from the nearest land': there, men could fully prove themselves. Yet the ideal of the universal man persists. It could be the promise implicit in automation and its gift of long-term leisure.

Sassall's desire to be universal cannot therefore be dismissed as a purely personal form of megalomania. He has an appetite for experience which keeps pace with his imagination and which has not been suppressed. It is the knowledge of the impossibility of satisfying any such appetite for new experience which kills the imagination of most people over thirty in our society.

Sassall is a fortunate exception and it is this which makes him seem in spirit – though not in appearance – much younger than he is. There are superficial aspects of him which are still like a student. For example, he enjoys dressing up in 'uniforms' for different activities and wearing them with all the casualness of the third-year expert: a sweater and stocking cap for working on the land in winter: a deer-stalker and laced leather leggings for shooting with his dog: an umbrella and homburg for funerals. When he has to read notes at a public meeting he *deliberately* looks over his glasses like a schoolmaster. If you met him outside his area, on

neutral ground, and if he didn't begin talking, you might
for one moment suppose that he was an actor.

He might have been one. In this way too he would
have played many roles. The desire to proliferate
the self into many selves may initially grow
from a tendency to exhibitionism. But for Sassall as
the doctor he is now, the motive is entirely transformed.
There can be no audience. It is only he who can
judge his own 'exhibition'. The motive now is
knowledge: knowledge almost in the Faustian sense.

The passion for knowledge is described by Browning
in his poem about Paracelsus – whose life story
was one of the tributaries to the later Faust legend.

> *I cannot feed on beauty for the sake*
> *Of beauty only, nor can drink in balm*
> *From lovely objects for their loveliness;*
> *My nature cannot lose her first imprint;*
> *I still must board and heap and class all truths*
> *With one ulterior purpose: I must know!*
> *Would God translate me to his throne, believe*
> *That I should only listen to his word*
> *To further my own aim!*

Sassall, unlike Paracelsus, is neither a theosophist nor
a *Magus*; he believes more in the science than in
the art of medicine.

'When people talk about doctors being artists, it's
nearly always due to the shortcomings of society.
In a better society, in a juster one, the doctor would
be much more of a pure scientist.'

Or:

'The essential tragedy of the human situation is not
knowing. Not knowing what we are or why we
are – for *certain*. But this doesn't lead me to religion.
Religion doesn't answer it.'

Yet this difference of emphasis is mostly an historical
one. At the time of Paracelsus sickness was thought
of as the scourge of God: and yet was welcomed
as a warning because it was finite whereas
hell was eternal. Suffering was the condition of the

earthly life: the only true relief was the life to
come. There is a striking contrast in medieval art
between the way animals and human beings
are depicted. The animals are free to be themselves,
sometimes horrific, sometimes beautiful. The
human beings are restrained and anxious. The animals
celebrate the present. The humans are all waiting
– waiting for the judgement which will decide the nature
of their immortality. At times it seems that some of
the artists envied the animals their mortality:
with that mortality went a freedom from the closed
system which reduced life here and now to a metaphor.
Medicine, such as it was, was also metaphorical.
When autopsies were performed and actually revealed to
the eye the false teachings of Galenic medicine,
the evidence was dismissed as accidental or
exceptional. Such was the strength of the system's
metaphors – and the impossibility, the irrelevance of any
medical science. Medicine was a branch of theology.
Little wonder that Paracelsus who came from
such a system and then challenged it in the name of
independent observation resorted sometimes to
mumbo-jumbo! Partly to give himself confidence, partly
for protection.

I am not, of course, implying that Sassall is an
historically comparable figure to Paracelsus.
But I suspect that he is in the same vocational tradition.
There are doctors who are craftsmen, who are
politicians, who are laboratory researchers, who are
ministers of mercy, who are businessmen, who
are hypnotists, etc. But there are also doctors who – like
certain Master Mariners – want to experience
all that is possible, who are driven by curiosity. But
'curiosity' is too small a word and 'the spirit of enquiry'
is too institutionalized. They are driven by the need
to know. The patient is their material. Yet to
them, more than to any doctor in any of the other
categories, the patient, in his totality, is for that very
reason sacred.

When patients are describing their conditions or
worries to Sassall, instead of nodding his head
or murmuring 'yes', he says again and again 'I know',
'I know'. He says it with genuine sympathy. Yet
it is what he says whilst he is waiting to know more.
He already knows what it is like to be this
patient in a certain condition: but he does not yet know
the full explanation of that condition, nor the
extent of his own power.

In fact no answer to these open questions will ever
satisfy him. Part of him is always waiting to
know more – at every surgery, on every visit, every
time the telephone rings. Like any Faust without the aid
of the devil, he is a man who suffers frequently from
a sense of anti-climax.

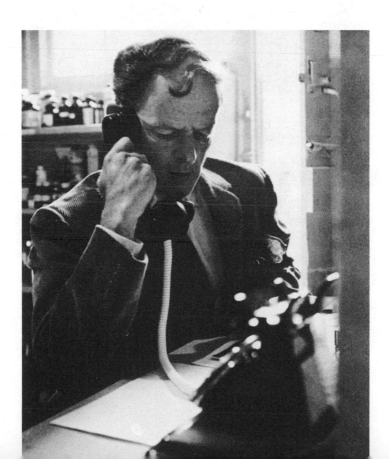

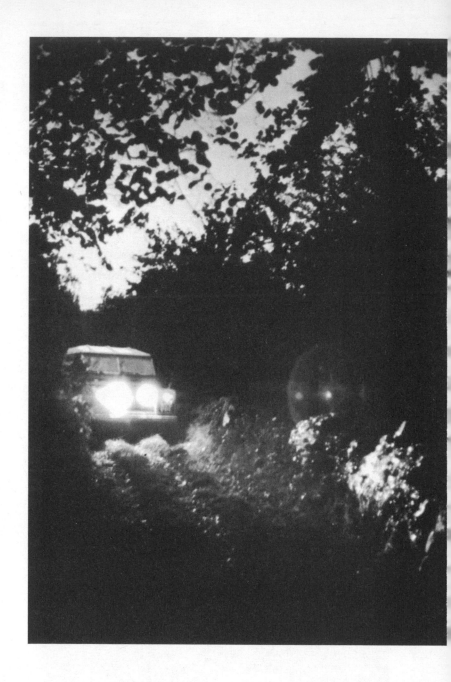

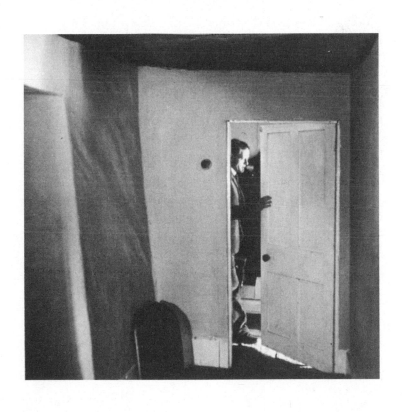

This is why he exaggerates when he tells stories about himself. In these stories he is nearly always in an absurd position: trying to take a film on deck when the waves break over him; getting lost in a city he doesn't know; letting a pneumatic drill run away with him. He stresses the disenchantment and deliberately makes himself a comic little man. Disguised in this way and forearmed against disappointment, he can then re-approach reality once more with the entirely un-comic purposes of mastering it, of understanding further. You can see this in the difference between his two eyes: his right eye knows what to expect – it can laugh, sympathize, be stern, mock itself, take aim: his left eye scarcely ever ceases considering the distant evidence and searching.

I say scarcely ever, but there is one exception. This is when he is occupied with some relatively minor surgical task. He may be setting a fracture in his surgery, or attending to one of his patients in the local hospital. On these occasions both eyes concentrate on the task in hand and a look of relief comes over his face. As soon as he takes his coat off, rolls up his sleeves, washes his hands, puts on gloves or a mask, this relief is apparent. It is as though his mind is wiped clean (hence the relief) in order to concentrate exclusively on the limited operation in hand. For a moment there is certainty. The job can be done well or badly: the distinction between the two is beyond dispute: and it must be done well.

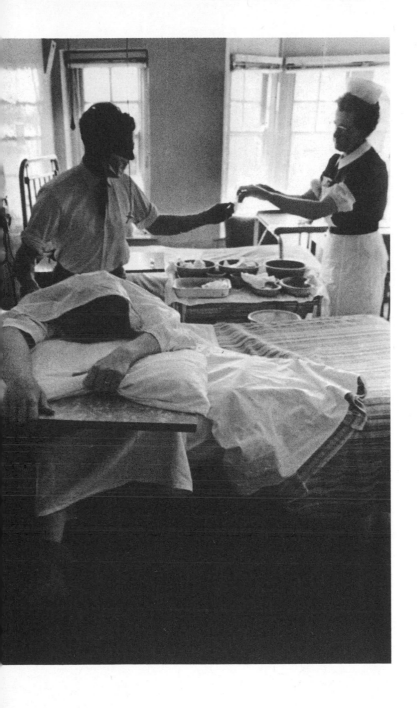

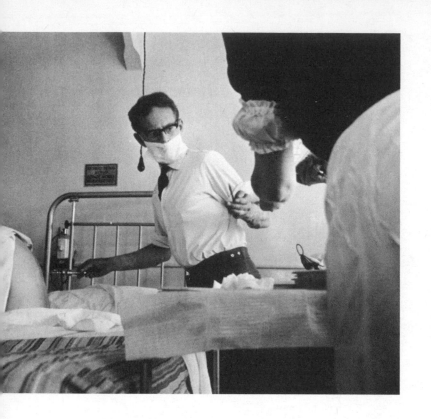

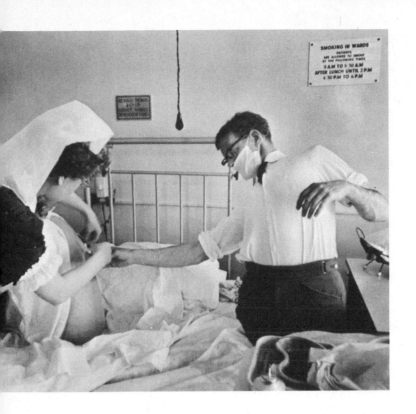

I saw a similar expression on the face of a farmer who
lives only a few miles from Sassall. This farmer is
mad about flying and owns a six-cylinder open-cockpit
Czech plane. His farm is not a large or particularly
prosperous one. Nor is he part of the gentry. He lives by
himself and likes speed. He keeps the plane under
an oak-tree in one of his fields. When we had driven the
sheep to the other end of the field, and I had
turned the prop and he and Jean Mohr were settled and
the engine was warm, he signalled to me to let go
of the tip of the wing – I was holding it for the plane
had no brakes – and at that moment, just before
they took off, although there was a gusty wind blowing
and the field was very rough and the take-off was
liable to be quite tricky, I saw exactly the same look of
relief pass over the farmer's unshaved, chunky,
middle-aged face. The problems now were limited to
aerodynamics and the functioning of a small
internal-combustion engine: the problem of prices,
mortgages, Monday's market, relations, reputation,
would all in a moment be beneath them.

The difference between the farmer and Sassall is that
the farmer would like to be able to spend all his
life blithely flying and gliding – or anyway believes that
he would; whereas Sassall needs his unsatisfied
quest for certainty and his uneasy sense of unlimited
responsibility.

So far I have tried to describe something of Sassall's
relationship with his patients. I have tried to show why
he is thought of as a good doctor, and how being
'a good doctor' answers some of his own needs. I have
suggested something of the mechanism by which
he cures others to cure himself. But all this has been on
an individual basis. We must now consider his
relationship to the local community as a whole. What do
his patients expect of him publicly when they are

not ill? And how does this relate to their
barely formulated expectations of fraternity within the
privacy of illness?

Sassall lives in one of the larger houses of the village.
He is well dressed. He drives a Land Rover for his
practice, and another car for his private use.
His children go to the local grammar school. Without
any doubt at all the part allotted him is that of
gentleman.

The area as a whole is economically depressed. There
are only a few large farms and no large-scale
industries. Fewer than half the men work on the land.
Most earn their living in small workshops,
quarries, a wood-processing factory, a jam factory, a
brickworks. They form neither a proletariat nor
a traditional rural community. They belong to the Forest
and in the surrounding districts they are invariably
known as 'the foresters'. They are suspicious,
independent, tough, poorly educated, low church. They
have something of the character once associated
with wandering traders like tinkers.

Sassall has done his best to modify the part of
gentleman allotted him, and has partly succeeded. He
leads almost no social life of his own – except in
the village with the villagers. It is when he is talking
with his few middle-class neighbours that one
is most aware of his own class background. This is
because they assume in conversation and attitude that he
shares their prejudices. With the 'foresters' he
seems like a foreigner who has become, by request, the
clerk of their own records.

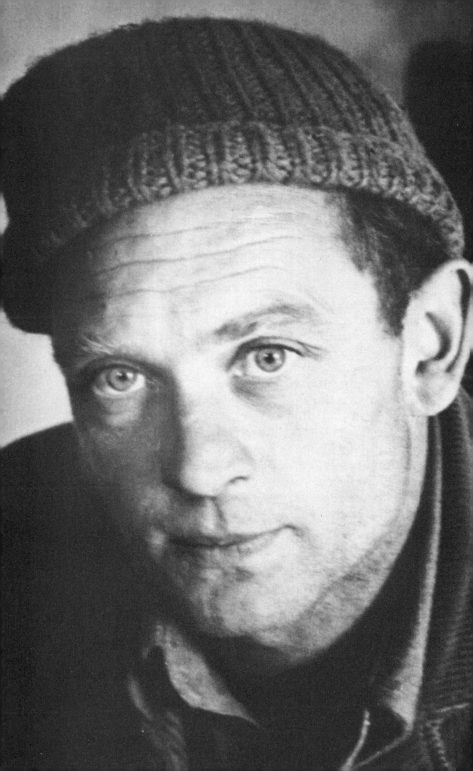

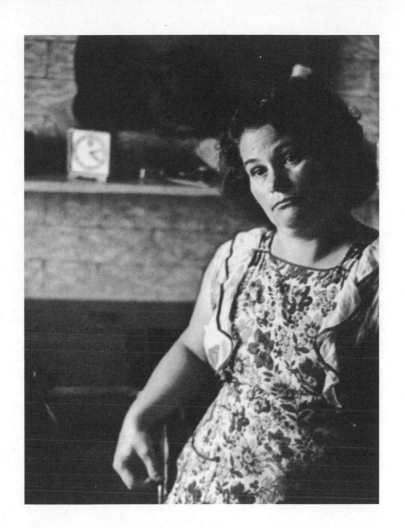

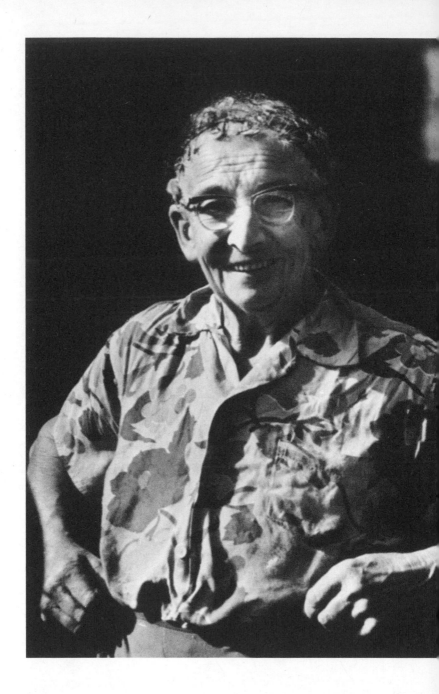

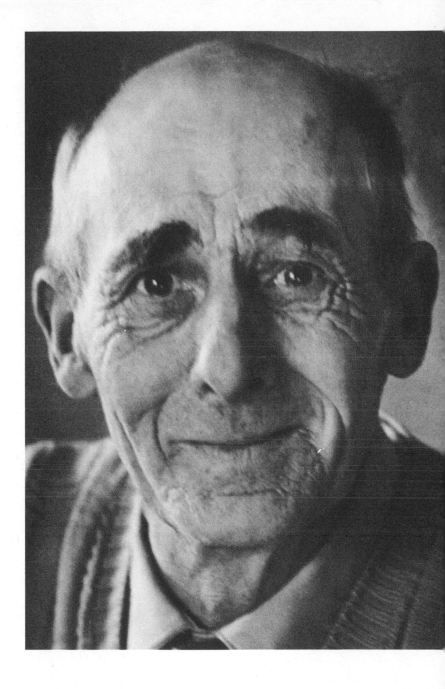

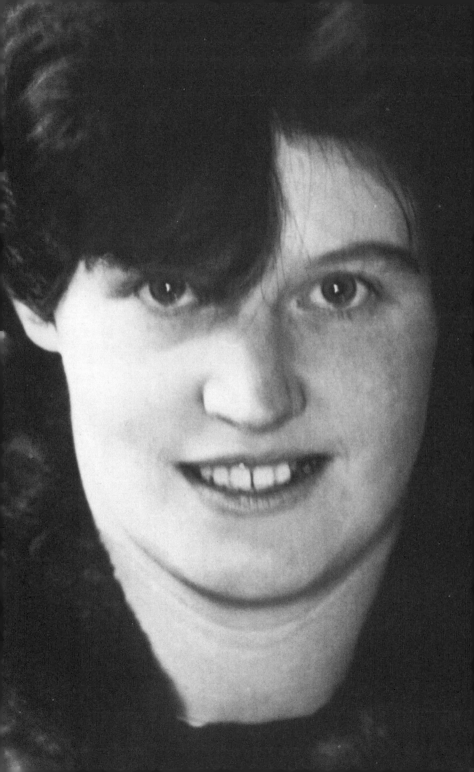

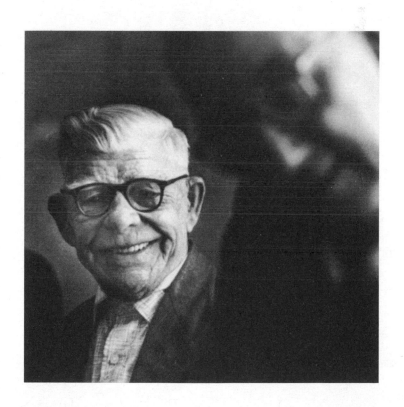

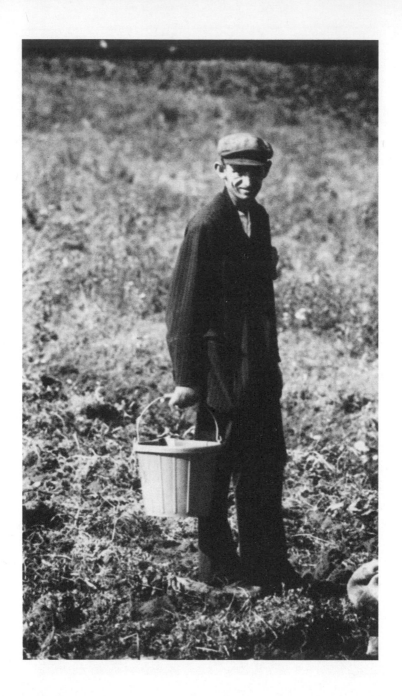

Let me try to explain what I mean by 'the clerk of the foresters' records'.

'Where you're different Doc is I know I can say Fuck You to your face if I want to.' Yet the speaker never has said Fuck You to Sassall.

'You're the laziest bitch I've ever come across,' says Sassall to the middle-aged woman draper whose day is now made. Yet only he can say this to her.

'What have you got on?' he asks about a menu at a factory canteen.

'Do you want to start at the top,' answers the girl at the counter pointing to her breasts, 'or at the bottom?' lifting her skirts up high. Yet she knows she is safe with the doctor.

Sassall has to a large extent liberated himself and the image of himself in the eyes of his patients from the conventions of social etiquette. He has done this by becoming unconventional. Yet the unconventional doctor is a traditional figure. Where Sassall perhaps is different is that traditionally the unconventionality has only allowed the doctor to swear at and shock his patients instead of vice versa. Sassall would like to think that anybody can say anything to him. But insofar as this is true, it confirms rather than denies his position of privilege. To your equals you cannot say anything: you learn very precisely the form and area of their tolerance. The theoretical freedom of address towards Sassall implies his authority, his special 'exemption', precisely because theoretically it is total. In practice anything unconventional which he says or which is said to him in public is a gesture – no more – against the idea that his authority is backed by the authority of society. It is the form of personal recognition he demands of his patients in exchange for the very different recognition he offers them.

In the village there is a medieval castle with a wide, deep
moat round it. This moat was used as a kind of
unofficial dump. It was overgrown with trees, bushes,
weeds, and full of stones, old wood, muck, gravel.
Five years ago Sassall had the idea of turning it into a
garden for the village. Tens of thousands of
man-hours of work would be involved. He formed a
'society' to occupy itself with the task and he
was elected chairman. The work was to be done in the
summer evenings and at week-ends whenever the
men of the village were free. Farmers lent
their machinery and tractors; a roadmaker brought his
bull-dozer along; somebody borrowed a crane.

Sassall himself worked hard on the project. If he
was not in the surgery and not out on a call, he could be
found in the moat most summer evenings. Now
the moat is a lawned garden with a fountain, roses,
shrubs and seats to sit on.

'Nearly all the planning of the work in the moat,' says
Sassall, 'was done by Ted, Harry, Stan, John, etc.,
etc. I don't mean they were better at doing the
work, better with their hands – they were that – but
they also had better ideas.'

Sassall was constantly involved in technical discussion
of these ideas with the men of the village. The
conversations over the weeks continued for hours. As a
result a social – as distinct from medical – intimacy
was established.

This might seem to be the obvious result of just
getting on with a job together. But it is not as simple or
as superficial as that. The job offers the possibility of
talking together, and finally the talk transcends the job.

The inarticulateness of the English is the subject of
many jokes and is often explained in terms of
puritanism, shyness as a national characteristic, etc. This
tends to obscure a more serious development.
There are large sections of the English working and
middle class who are inarticulate as the result
of wholesale cultural deprivation. They are deprived of

the means of translating what they know into thoughts which they can think.* They have no examples to follow in which words clarify experience. Their spoken proverbial traditions have long been destroyed: and, although they are literate in the strictly technical sense, they have not had the opportunity of discovering the existence of a written cultural heritage.

Yet it is more than a question of literature. Any general culture acts as a mirror which enables the individual to recognize himself – or at least to recognize those parts of himself which are socially permissible. The culturally deprived have far fewer ways of recognizing themselves. A great deal of their experience – especially emotional and introspective experience – has to remain *unnamed* for them. Their chief means of self-expression is consequently through action: this is one of the reasons why the English have so many 'do-it-yourself' hobbies. The garden or the work bench becomes the nearest they have to a means of satisfactory introspection.

The easiest – and sometimes the only possible – form of conversation is that which concerns or describes action: that is to say action considered as technique or as procedure. It is then not the experience of the speakers which is discussed but the nature of an entirely exterior mechanism or event – a motor-car engine, a football match, a draining system or the workings of some committee. Such subjects, which preclude anything directly personal, supply the content of most of the conversations being carried on by men over twenty-five at any given moment in England today. (In the case of the young, the force of their own appetites saves them from such depersonalization.)

* My novel *Corker's Freedom* (New York: Vintage International, 1995) attempts to illuminate this situation.

Yet there is warmth in such conversation and friendships can be made and sustained by it. The very intricacy of the subjects seems to bring the speakers close together. It is as though the speakers bend over the subject to examine it in precise detail, until, bending over it, their heads touch. Their shared expertise becomes a symbol of shared experience. When friends recall another friend who is dead or absent, they recall how he always maintained that a front-wheel drive was safer: and in their memory this now acquires the value of an intimacy.

The area in which Sassall practises is one of extreme cultural deprivation, even by English standards. And it was only by working with many of the men of the village and coming to understand something of their techniques that he could qualify for their conversation. They then came to share a language which was a metaphor for the rest of their common experience.

Sassall would like to believe that the metaphor implies that they talk as equals: the more so because within the range of the language the villagers mostly know far more than he. Yet they do not talk as equals.

Sassall is accepted by the villagers and foresters as a man who, in the full sense of the term, lives with them. Face to face with him, whatever the circumstances, there is no need for shame or complex explanations: he will understand even when their own community as a whole will not or cannot. (Most unmarried girls who become pregnant come to him straightway without any prevarication.) Insofar as he is feared at all, it is by a few older patients in whom a little of the traditional fear of the doctor still persists. (This traditional fear, apart from being a rational fear of the consequences of illness, is also an irrational fear of the consequences of making their secret but outrageous and insistent demand for fraternity to doctors who always behave and are treated as their superiors.)

In general his patients think of Sassall as 'belonging' to their community. He represents no outside interest – in such an area any outside interest suggests exploitation. He is trusted. Yet this is not the same thing as saying that he is thought of or treated as an equal.

It is evident to everybody that he is privileged. This is accepted as a matter of course: nobody resents or questions it. It is part of his being the kind of doctor he is. The privilege does not concern his income, his car or his house: these are merely amenities which make it possible for him to do his job. And if through them he enjoys a little more comfort than the average, it is still not a question of privilege, for certainly he has earned a right to that comfort.

He is privileged because of the way he can think and can talk! If the estimate of his privilege was strictly logical, it would include the fact of his education and his medical training. But that was a long time ago, whereas the evidence of the way he thinks – not purely medically but in general – is there every time he is there. It is why the villagers talk to him, why they tell him the local news, why they listen, why they wonder whether his unusual views are right, why some say 'He's a wonderful doctor but not what you'd expect', and why some middle-class neighbours call him a crack-pot.

The villagers do not consider him privileged because they find his thinking so impressive. It is the style of his thinking which they immediately recognize as different from theirs. They depend upon common-sense and he does not.

It is generally thought that common-sense is practical. It is practical only in a short-term view. Common-sense declares that it is foolish to bite the hand that feeds you. But it is foolish only up to the moment when you realize that you might be fed very much better. In the long-term view common-sense is passive because it is based on the acceptance of an outdated view of the possible. The body of common-sense has to accrue too slowly. All its propositions have to be proved so many times before they can become unquestionable, i.e. traditional. When they become traditional they gain oracular authority. Hence the strong element of *superstition* always evident in 'practical' common-sense.

Common-sense is part of the home-made ideology of those who have been deprived of fundamental learning, of those who have been kept ignorant. This ideology is compounded from different sources: items that have survived from religion, items of empirical knowledge, items of protective scepticism, items culled for comfort from the superficial learning that *is* supplied. But the point is that common-sense can never teach itself, can never advance beyond its own limits, for as soon as the lack of fundamental learning has been made good, all items become questionable and the whole function of common-sense is destroyed. Common-sense can only exist as a category insofar as it can be distinguished from the spirit of enquiry, from philosophy.

Common-sense is essentially *static*. It belongs to the ideology, of those who are socially passive, never understanding what or who has made their situation as it is. But it represents only a part – and often a small part – of their character. These same people say or do many things which are an affront to their own common-sense. And when they justify something by saying 'It's only common-sense', this is frequently an apology for denying or betraying some of their deepest feelings or instincts.

Sassall accepts his innermost feelings and intuitions as clues. His own self is often his most promising starting-point. His aim is to find what may be hidden in others:

'I don't find it hard to express uncensored thoughts or sentiments but when I do, it keeps on occurring

to me that this is a form of self-indulgence. That sounds
somewhat pompous, but still. At least it makes me
realize and understand why patients thank me so
profusely for merely listening: they too are apologizing
for what they think – wrongly – is their self-indulgence.'

Using his own mortality as another starting-point
he needs to find references of hope or possibility in an
almost unimaginable future.

'I'm encouraged by the fact that the molecules of
this table and glass and plant are rearranged to make you
or me, and that the bad things are perhaps badly
arranged molecules and therefore capable maybe of
reorganization one day.'

Yet however fanciful his speculations, he returns to
measure them by the standards of actual knowledge
to date. And then from this measurement begins
to speculate again.

'You never know *for certain* about anything. This
sounds falsely modest and trite, but it's the honest truth.
Most of the time you are right and you do *appear*
to know, but every now and then the rules seem to get
broken and then you realize how lucky you have
been on the occasions when *you think you have known* and
have been proved correct.'

He never stops speculating, testing, comparing.
The more open the question the more it interests him.

Such a way of thinking demands the right to
be theoretical and to be concerned with generalizations.
Yet theory and generalizations belong by their nature
to the cities or the distant capital where the big general
decisions are always made. Furthermore, to arrive
at general decisions and theories one needs to travel in
order to gain experience. Nobody travels from
the Forest. So nobody in the Forest has either the power
or the means to theorize. They are 'practical' people.

It may seem surprising to place so much emphasis on
geographic isolation and distances when England is
so small a country. Yet the subjective feeling
of remoteness has little to do with mileage. It is a

reaction to economic power. Monopoly – with its
mounting tendency to centralization – has even
turned what were once large, vital towns, like Bolton or
Rochdale or Wigan, into remote backwaters. And
in a country area, where the average level of political
consciousness is very low, all decision-making
which is not practical, all theory, seems to most of the
local inhabitants to be the privilege and prerogative
of distant policy-makers. The intellectual – and
this is why they are so suspicious of him – seems
to be part of the apparatus of the State which controls
them. Sassall is trusted because he lives with them.
But his way of thinking could only have been
acquired elsewhere. All theory-makers have cast at least
one eye on the seat of power. And that is a privilege
the foresters have never known.

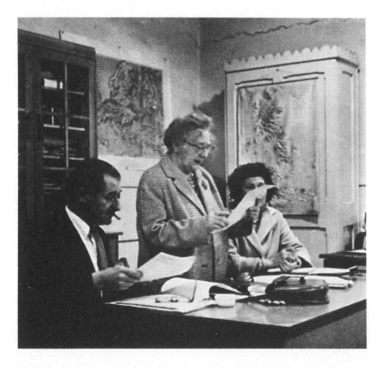

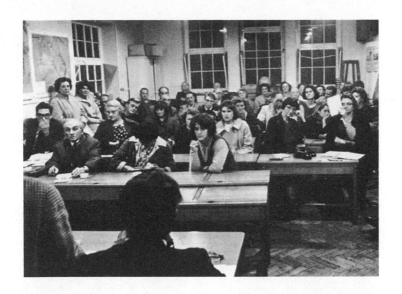

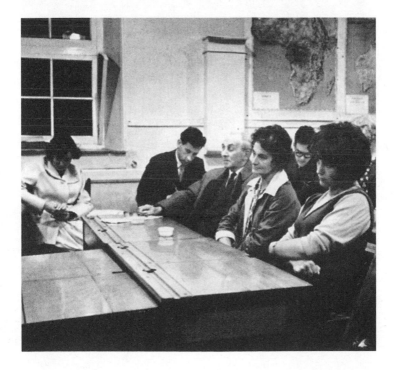

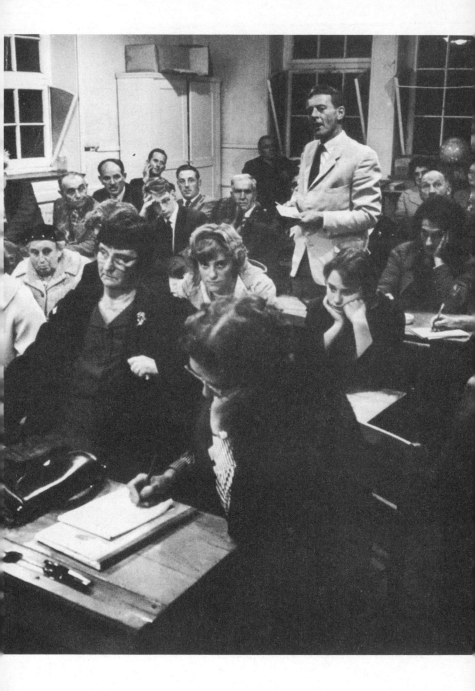

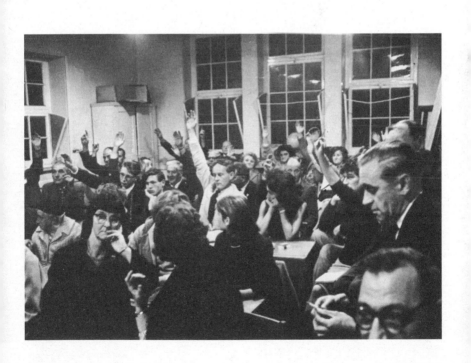

There is another reason why they sense that Sassall's
way of thinking is a privilege, but as a reason it
is less rational. Once it might have been considered
magical. He confesses to fear without fear.
He finds all impulses natural – or understandable.
He remembers what it is like to be a child. He
has no respect for any title as such. He can enter into
other people's dreams or nightmares. He can lose
his temper and then talk about the true
reasons, as opposed to the excuse, for why he did
so. His ability to do such things connects him
with aspects of experience which have to be either
ignored or denied by common-sense. Thus his 'licence'
challenges the prisoner in every one of his listeners.

There is probably only one other man in the area
whose mode of thinking is comparable. But this man is
a writer and a recluse. Nobody around him is aware
of how he thinks. There are clergymen and
schoolmasters and engineers, but they all use the syntax
of common-sense: it is only their vocabulary which
is different because they need to refer to God,
O-levels, or stresses in metal. Sassall's privilege seems
locally unique.

The attitude of the villagers and foresters to Sassall's
privilege is complex. He has got a good brain, they
say, why, with a brain like this – and then,
remembering that he belongs to them, they realize that
his choice of their remote country practice again
implies a kind of privilege: the privilege of
his indifference to success. But now his privilege
becomes to some extent their privilege. They are proud
of him and at the same time protective about him:
as though his choice suggested that a good brain
can also be a kind of weakness. They often look at him
quite anxiously. Yet they are not, I think, so proud
of him as a doctor – they know he is a good doctor but
they do not know how rare or common that is –
rather, they are proud of his way of thinking, of his
mind, which has mysteriously allowed him to choose to

stay with them. Without being directly influenced
by it, they make his way of thinking theirs by giving
it a local function.

He does more than treat them when they are ill; he is
the objective witness of their lives. They seldom
refer to him as a witness. They only think of him when
some practical circumstance brings them together.
He is in no way a final arbiter. That is why I chose the
rather humble word *clerk*: the clerk of their records.

He is qualified to be this precisely because of his
privilege. If the records are to be as complete as possible
– and who does not at times dream of the impossible
ideal of being totally recorded? – the records must
be related to the world at large, and they must include
what is hidden, even what is hidden within the
protagonists themselves.

Some may now assume that he has taken over
the role of the parish priest or vicar. Yet this is not so.
He is not the representative of an all-knowing,
all-powerful being. He is their own representative. His
records will never be offered to any higher judge.
He keeps the records so that, from time to time, they
can consult them themselves. The most frequent
opening to a conversation with him, if it is
not a professional consultation, are the words 'Do you
remember when . . .?' He represents them,
becomes their objective (as opposed to subjective)
memory, because he represents their lost possibility of
understanding and relating to the outside world,
and because he also represents some of what they know
but cannot think.

This is what I meant by his being the requested
clerk of their records. It is an honorary position.
He is seldom called upon to officiate. But it has its exact
if unstated meaning.   ϑ

I am very well aware that there is a certain clumsiness in my metaphorical devices. And what do they matter? On the one hand a sociological survey of medical country practice might be more useful: and on the other hand various statistical analyses of the degree of satisfaction expressed among patients after different forms of treatment might be more revealing. I do not for one moment deny the usefulness of such exercises – and indeed have drawn upon many of their findings whilst preparing this essay. But what I am trying to define here are relations which cannot yet be reached by a question-and-answer analysis.

What I am saying about Sassall and his patients is subject to the danger which accompanies any imaginative effort. At certain times my own subjectivity may distort. At no time can I prove what I am saying. I can only claim that after years of observation of the subject I believe that what I am saying, despite my clumsiness, reveals a significant part of the social reality of the small area in question, and a large part of the psychological reality of Sassall's life. The greatest stumbling-block to accepting this is the false view that what people cannot express is always simple because they are simple. We like to retain such a view because it confirms our own bogus sense of articulate individuality, and because it saves us from thinking about the extraordinarily complex convergence of philosophical traditions, feelings, half-realized ideas, atavistic instincts, imaginative intimations, which lie behind the simplest hope or disappointment of the simplest person.

To a large extent Sassall has achieved his ideal. As much as a man can on land, dealing with illness and not the sea, and living in the middle of the twentieth century, he has achieved a position which is comparable to that of a master of a schooner.

He has his relative autonomy and his solitary responsibilities. (Unlike most G.P.s, he has access to

ninety per cent of his hospitalized patients,
because all but complex major surgery cases go to the
local town hospital at which he is one of the
house doctors.) He deals with all emergencies which
arise – from serious accidents in the quarries or
at harvesting time in the fields, to the despair of a young
woman who wants to kill her illegitimate baby or
the slow suffering and eventual collapse of a retired vicar
who has lost his faith. He is trusted, almost without
question.

It is true that his attitude to the individual patient, far
from being based on explicit authority, is based
on answering an unmade demand for fraternity, but this
fraternity is *not* mutual: it is an imaginative projection
on Sassall's part, as true, but also as artificial as a
work of art: nobody fraternally recognizes Sassall: and
this makes him the commander.

His position as 'clerk of the records' not only
means that, more than any other man, he knows the
continuing history of the area; it also attributes to him
the power to comprehend and realize for the
community. To some extent he thinks and speaks what
the community feels and incoherently knows. To
some extent he is the growing force (albeit very slow) of
their self-consciousness.

Lastly, the area, because it is backward and depressed,
is subject to the minimum of direct influence from
outside. Its condition is entirely dependent upon what
happens and what is decided elsewhere. But very
few people, very few ideas – except the ready-to-wear
ones of the misused mass media – arrive to
challenge Sassall's hegemony.

What is the price of Sassall's achievement?

I do not propose to discuss all the daily irritations
and inconveniences of a G.P.'s life. This can
safely be left to representatives of the doctors themselves.
Some of their grievances are real enough. But the
general tone of them is the result of fear and

resentment at the sensed but not fully understood fact that the nineteenth-century status and categories of the medical profession are becoming obsolete.

Sassall is not really alarmed by this, for he has established his own special position. As a result of this special position, however, he has to face, far more nakedly than many doctors, the suffering of his patients and the frequent inadequacy of his ability to help them. ϑ

It is generally assumed that doctors take a professional view of suffering and that the process of professional insulation begins in their second year as medical students when they first start dissecting the human body. This is true. But the question is far deeper than overcoming any physical revulsion at the sight of blood or guts. Later, other factors are an aid to their self-protection. Doctors use a second, technical, entirely unemotional language. Frequently, they need to act quickly and to carry out complicated manual tasks which demand exclusive concentration. Increasing specialization encourages an increasingly scientific view of illness. (In the eighteenth century and earlier the doctor was often thought of as a cynic: a cynic is by definition a man who assumes a scientific 'objectivity' to which he has no claim.) The sheer number of their cases discourages self-identification with any individual patient.

Yet, however true this may be, the suffering which certain doctors witness may be more of a strain than is generally admitted. This is so with Sassall. He is a man of extreme self-control. Nevertheless, when he was unaware of my presence, I saw him weep, walking across a field away from a house where a young patient was dying. Perhaps he was blaming himself for things done or left undone. He would transform his pain into a sense of painful responsibility, for that is his character.

But his sensibility is not just the consequence of
his character: it is equally the consequence of
his position and the way he practises. He never separates
an illness from the total personality of the patient
– in this sense, he is the opposite of a specialist. He does
not believe in maintaining his imaginative distance:
he must come close enough to recognize the
patient fully. Although he has about 2,000 patients, he
is aware of how they are all inter-related – and
not only in the family sense – so that the numbers
seldom acquire a statistical objectivity for him. Most
important of all, he considers that it is his duty to try to
treat at least certain forms of unhappiness. He
very seldom sends a patient to mental hospital for he
considers it a kind of abandonment.

What is the effect of facing, trying to understand,
hoping to overcome the extreme anguish of
other persons five or six times a week? I do not speak
now of physical anguish, for that can usually
be relieved in a matter of minutes. I speak of the
anguish of dying, of loss, of fear, of loneliness, of being
desperately beside oneself, of the sense of futility.

One aspect of the confrontations seems to me to be
important and not much discussed, and so the
reader must forgive me if I concentrate on this and
ignore others.

Anguish has its own time-scale. What separates the
anguished person from the unanguished is a
barrier of time: a barrier which intimidates the
imagination of the latter.

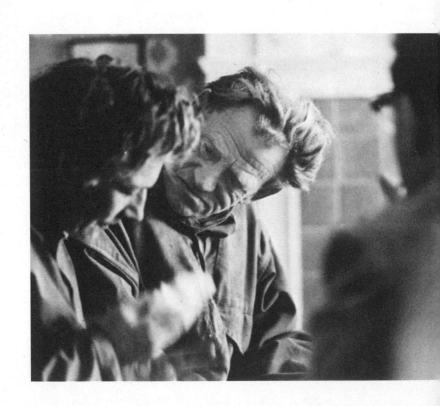

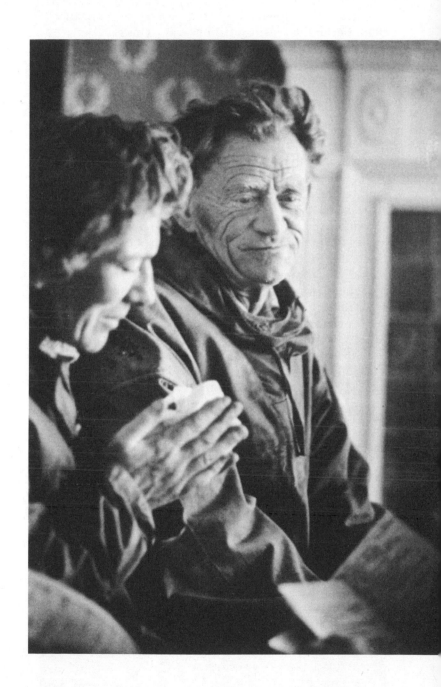

A man or a woman who is sobbing reminds one of a child, but in the most disturbing way. This is partly because of the particular social convention which discourages adults (and particularly men) from breaking into tears but permits children to do so. Yet this is by no means the whole explanation. There is a physical resemblance between a sobbing figure and a child. The 'bearing' of the adult falls away and his movements are limited to certain very primitive ones. The centre of the body once again seems to be the mouth: as though the mouth were simultaneously the place of pain and the only way by which consolation might be taken in. There is a loss of the control of the hands which again can only clench or paw. The whole body tends towards a foetal position. There are good physiological and psychological reasons for all this: but we can observe the similarity without knowing them. And why is the similarity so disturbing? Once more I believe the explanation goes further than our sense of convention or compassion. In some way the similarity, once established, is brutally denied. The sobbing man is not like a child. The child cries to protest. The man cries to himself. It may even be that by crying again like a child he somehow believes that he will regain the ability to recover like a child. Yet that is impossible.

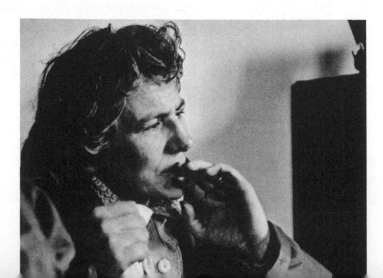

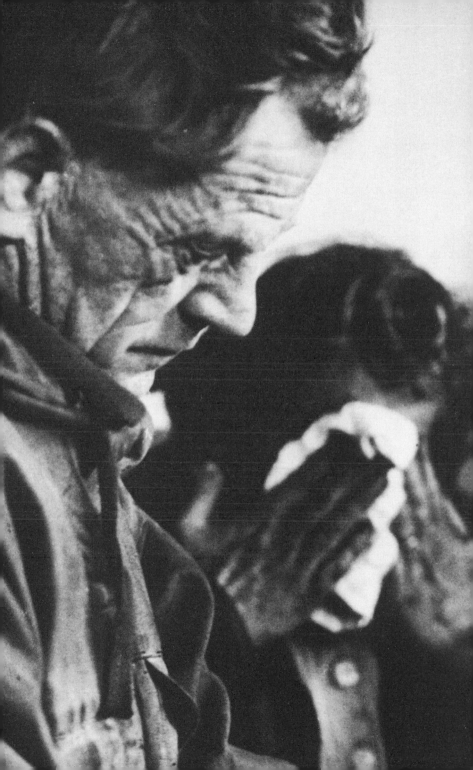

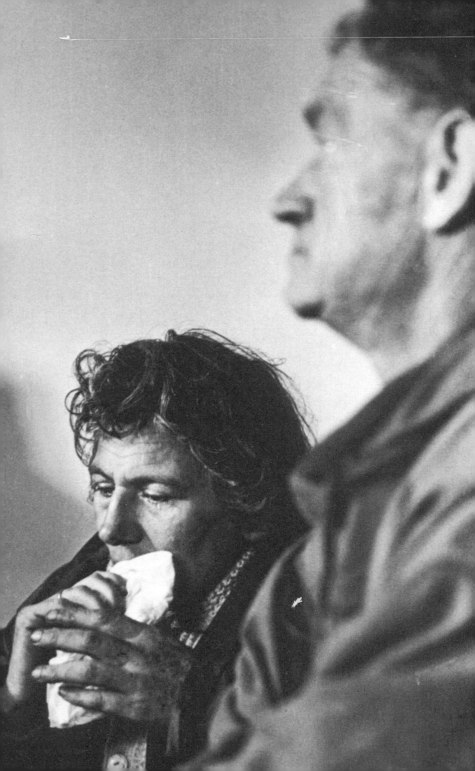

Anguish need not necessarily involve weeping. It may
be composed more bitterly in hatred, vengeance
or in that half-mocking anticipation of cruelty with
which the desperate sometimes await their own
destruction. But all anguish, whatever its expression of
cause and whether it is rational or neurotic,
returns the sufferer to a childhood which increases his
despair. Or at least that is what I believe as a
result of my own observation and introspection.

It is a platitude that as we grow older time seems to
pass more quickly. The remark is usually made
nostalgically. But we seldom consider the contrary effect
of the same process – the elongation of time as it
must affect the young and very young. The
young themselves can say little about it, because they
only have a standard of judgement when they
become aware of time changing its pace and by then it's
too late for any direct evidence. If we knew how
long a night or a day was to a child, we might
understand a great deal more about childhood. Could it
not be that the deeply formative nature of early
childhood experience is due not only to the force of its
impact (a force measured by the child's relative
weakness) but also to the fact that by the child's own
reckoning the experiences continue for so long?
It may be that, subjectively, a childhood is at least equal
in length to the rest of a lifetime. The phenomenon
of old people, when their daily practical preoccupations
are reduced to a minimum, remembering more
and more clearly more and more about their childhood
may confirm this; subjectively, their childhood was
perhaps most of their life.

Yet why should time seem to change its pace? What
is the difference between a child and an adult in
this respect? Sartre in his first novel* offers a clue.

* *Nausea.* Jean-Paul Sartre (translated by Robert Baldick)
(Harmondsworth: Penguin, 1965).
The novel was first published in France in 1938.

The book as a whole is partly concerned with a similar and parallel problem: how to achieve a sense of adventure given a full awareness of the nature of time. This is how he describes the habitual life of the adult.

When you are living, nothing happens. The settings change, people come in and go out, that's all. There are never any beginnings. Days are tacked on to days without rhyme or reason, it is an endless, monotonous addition. Now and then you do a partial sum: you say: I've been travelling for three years, I've been at Bouville for three years. There isn't any end either: you never leave a woman, a friend, a town in one go. And then everything is like everything else: Shanghai, Moscow, Algiers, are all the same after a couple of weeks. Occasionally – not very often – you take bearings, you realize that you're living with a woman, mixed up in some dirty business. Just for an instant. After that, the procession starts again, you begin adding up the hours and days once more. Monday, Tuesday, Wednesday. April, May, June. 1924, 1925, 1926.

Sartre contrasts this 'living' with the occasional 'feeling of adventure'. This feeling need have nothing to do with exciting events. It is a form of heightened awareness giving a sensation of order – and therefore of meaning – to the very fact and limitations of existence.

This feeling of adventure definitely doesn't come from events: I have proved that. It's rather the way in which moments are linked together. This, I think, is what happens: all of a sudden you feel that time is passing, that each moment leads to another moment, this one to yet another and so on; that each moment destroys itself and that it's no use trying to hold back, etc., etc., and then you attribute this property to the events which appear to you *in* the moments; you extend to the contents what appertains to the form. . . .
If I remember rightly, they call that the irreversibility of time. The feeling of adventure would simply be that of the irreversibility of time. But why don't we always have it?

The irreversibility of time is something that young children are well aware of, although the concept could mean nothing to them. They live with it. There are no inevitable repetitions in childhood. 'Monday, Tuesday, Wednesday. April, May, June. 1924, 1925, 1926' represents the antithesis of their experience. Nothing is bound to repeat itself. Which, incidentally, is one of the reasons why children ask to be reassured that some things will be repeated. 'And tomorrow I will get up and have breakfast?' Gradually after the age of about six, they can answer the question for themselves and they begin to expect and depend upon cycles of events; but even then their unit of measurement is so small – their impatience, if you wish to call it that, is so great – that the foreseen still seems too far off to qualify the present to any important degree: their attention still remains on the present in which things constantly appear for the first time and are constantly being lost for ever.

One of the most widespread adult illusions is the belief in second chances. Children, until they are otherwise persuaded or bribed by adults, know that they do not exist. Their necessary self-abandonment to experience makes it impossible for them to entertain such an idea. The adult belief in them is a double buffer against experience. Not only is everyone given countless second chances, but the uniqueness of every event is blurred over, if not destroyed. And so, as time goes on, or rather fails to go on, we can tentatively propose that the world has become familiar with us, even that the world on the basis of past events is our debtor. Children have no need for such protection.

They have no need for it because their own opportunities seem to stretch further than they can imagine. Their own time is endless. They are constantly experiencing a sense of loss: it is the prerequisite, as Sartre points out, of a sense of adventure. Every parting, however trivial, the end of any game or event,

represents a final loss which no repetition will
mend. Sometimes they need to protest: then they cry out
in the hope that the loss can be postponed, or in
true regret for what has gone. I say *true* regret because it
is the thing lost which remains the centre of their
attention: not, as frequently with adults, their
own imagined state of deprivation in the future. Their
sense of loss is bounded by the next event or
interest. Young children have an almost insatiable
appetite for 'the next thing'. The next is needed to take
the place of what has irrevocably gone.

There is another reason why young children recover
from total loss so quickly. Nothing fortuitous
happens in a child's world. There are no accidents.
Everything is connected with everything else
and everything can be explained by everything else.*
(The structure of their world is similar to that
of magic.) Thus for a young child a loss is never
meaningless, absurd – and, above all, unnecessary. For a
young child everything that happens is a necessity.

When we suffer anguish we return to early childhood
because that is the period in which we first learnt to
suffer the experience of total loss. It was more
than that. It was the period in which we suffered more
total losses than in all the rest of our life put
together. Even supposing that no neurotic pattern still
forces us to react as we once reacted on some forgotten
but terrible occasion as a child, we are bound to
refer ourselves back to that period, for in the
intervening years we have only rarely and perhaps never
grasped, as we had to grasp continually as children,
the iron irreversibility of events.

And yet we are not children even when we
suffer again in this way. Above all, we can be aware, as
children cannot, of the arbitrariness of our
condition. What Sartre calls its gratuitousness.

* See Jean Piaget, *Language and Thought of the Child:* 3rd edn
(London: Routledge & Kegan Paul, 1959).

I mean that, by definition, existence is not necessity. To exist is simply *to be there*; what exists appears, lets itself be *encountered*, but you can never *deduce* it. There are people, I believe, who have understood that. Only they have tried to overcome this contingency by inventing a necessary, casual being. But no necessary being can explain existence: contingency is not an illusion, an appearance which can be dissipated; it is absolute, and consequently perfect gratuitousness. Everything is gratuitous, that park, this town, and myself. When you realize that, it turns your stomach over and everything starts floating about, as it did the other evening at the Rendez-vous Des Cheminots; that is the Nausea. . .

A depressed or bereaved forester obviously does not think like a professional philosopher. But he can see the forest, or the gas-stove in the downstairs room, or the newspapers piled under the dresser in the same light as Sartre describes here. It is almost a question of the light – or rather of how the mind interprets the light. It is a light which objectifies everything and confirms nothing. No child ever sees such a light. It is as different from the light in which a child sees the forest or the kitchen as is darkness.

I wonder whether I begin to make myself clear. Anguish arises from a sense of irreparable loss. (The loss may be real or imaginary.) This loss is added to all the other losses sustained during one's life: these other losses represent the *absence* of what one might otherwise have turned to for consolation on the occasion of this one, the most recent and final of all. Most of these other losses were suffered in childhood – for that is the nature of childhood. Thus the experience of loss tends to return, redeliver one to one's childhood. If the experience is partly or wholly neurotic, the return to childhood is actually part of the experience. If the experience is not neurotic, it is the sense of helplessness which leads one back. This helplessness – equally present in neurotic cases – changes one's sense of time. It is a helplessness in face of

the real or imagined irreversibility of what
has happened. Such awareness of irreversibility slows
down time. Moments can 'seem like years' because, like
a child, one feels that everything has changed for
ever. The notion of repetition is suddenly removed from
the reality of time. In the case of young children
this can amount to a form of heightened awareness and
is indeed the secret of much of their sense of
adventure. But this is because they are able to explain
and justify – at least on one level – everything that
happens, every loss included. By contrast the
anguished adult suffers the conviction that what has
happened is absurd; or at the best, is without sufficient
meaning. That is to say the meaning which remains
cannot possibly balance what has been lost. Consequently
the man or woman in anguish is trapped in the
time-scale of childhood without a child's protection,
suffering a uniquely adult agony.

Sassall meets anguished patients on his rounds – the
close relatives of the dying, those who are ill and
want to die, the immobilized who are made desperate
by a kind of claustrophobic fear of their own bodies,
the insanely jealous, the lonely who try to kill themselves,
the hysterics; sometimes he is able to reach them:
sometimes it is obvious that he never will. In
the evenings after supper he has long appointments
lasting an hour with patients whom he believes
he can help through psychotherapy. They suffer their
crises with him and these crises too can mount
to the pitch of anguish.

The psychologist G. M. Carstairs, writing from the
comparatively detached point of view of a teaching
professor, in no way underestimates the stress of
such encounters.

To encounter a fellow human being in a state of despair
compels one to share, at least in imagination, his
elemental problems: Is there any meaning in life? Is there
any point in his staying alive?

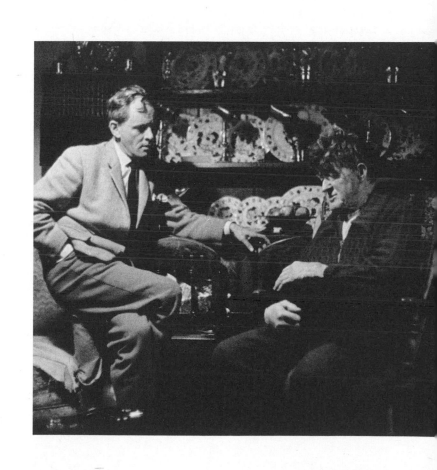

I believe, however, that the questions tend to present themselves to Sassall in terms of the experience of time. The elemental problem becomes: What is the value of the moment?

It is as though time became the equivalent of Conrad's sea: the sickness the equivalent of the weather. It is time which can promise 'the peace of God' and which can lash and destroy with 'unimaginable' fury. Again I am forced to use what may be a clumsy metaphor in the attempt to define a hidden, subjective experience – the generalized impact on a doctor's imagination of the suffering which he meets almost daily and which cannot be settled by writing prescriptions.

Sassall attends all the midwifery cases in his practice – is present at almost every birth. He is also present at most deaths. He is continually being reminded of how much difference a moment can make and of how irreversible, how carefully prepared the process which leads up to that moment is. To some degree he can interfere with the process. He can speed it up, he can slow it down, he can 'play for time'. But he cannot turn the sea into dry land.

Patients, when their illness has been given a name, usually ask next: And how long will it take? How long will it be before . . .? How long? How long? And the doctor replies that he cannot promise but . . . He can appear to be the controller of time, as, on occasions, the mariner appears to rule the sea. But both doctor and mariner know this to be an illusion.

All doctors are more than usually aware of death – though some do their best to hide the metaphysical fact by thinking only in terms of the physiological stages of dying. In the human imagination death and the passing of time are indissolubly linked: each moment that passes brings us nearer to our death: and our death, if it can be measured at all, is measured by that apparent eternity of existence which must continue after and without us.

This may help to explain Sassall's preoccupation with time. What is the value of the moment *sub specie aeternitatis*? But the confrontation with anguish is even more important. The anguished are trapped in a moment which is born of all that has happened to them. Faced with the rigid irreversibility of events – so terrible for all who are unprepared, and none can be fully prepared – it is their experience which bends in a circle: unable to catch time by the tail, they chase their own, revolving in one moment blindly through all their life. How much then can a moment contain?

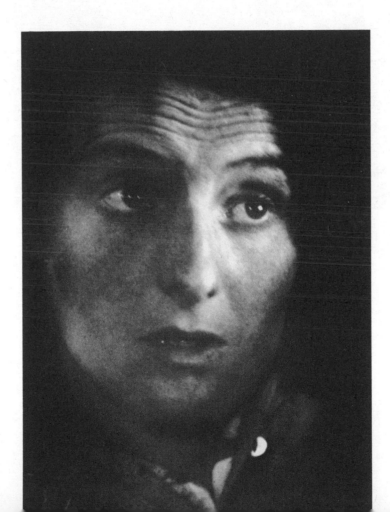

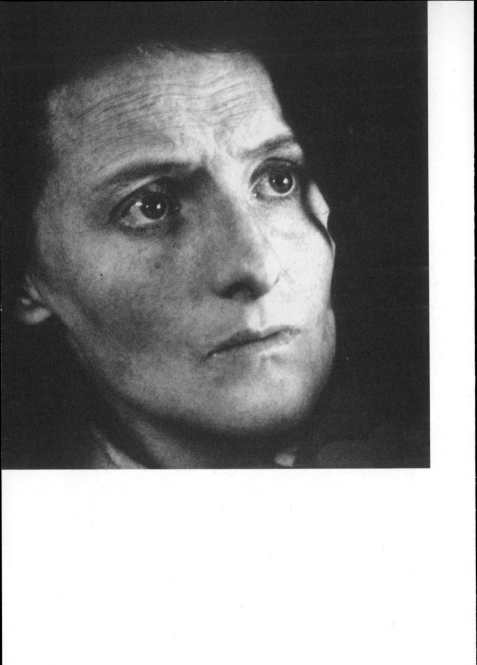

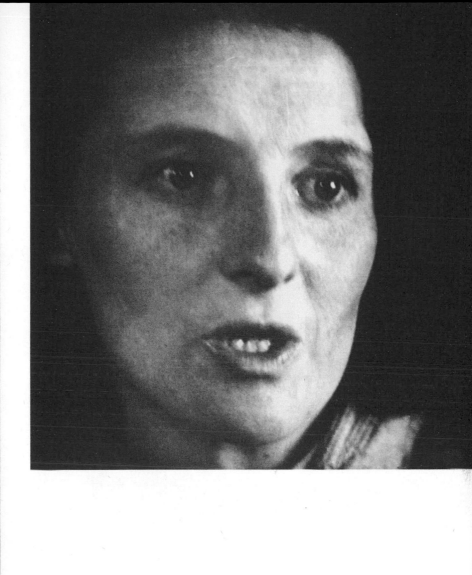

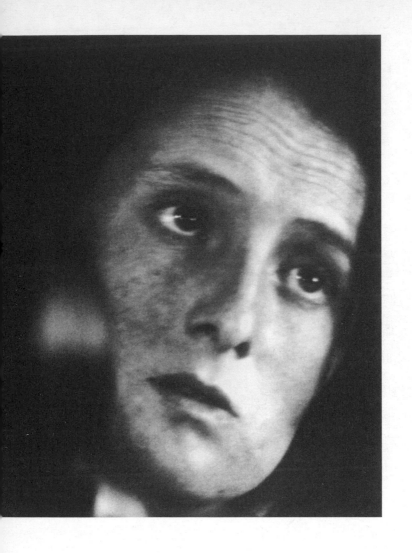

And how can one moment be compared to another person's experience of the same moment? Often it seems almost incredible that Sassall putting out a hand to touch a patient finds the patient there, coexisting.

The objective co-ordinates of time and space, which are necessary to fix a presence, are relatively stable. But the subjective experience of time is liable to be so grossly distorted – above all by suffering – that it becomes, both to the sufferer and to any person partially identifying himself with the sufferer, extremely difficult to correlate with time proper.

Sassall not only has to make this correlation, he also has to correlate the patient's subjective experience of time with his own subjective experience. When he has left the patient and is turning the Land Rover round, preparing to drive off, he may suddenly glimpse out of the corner of his mind's eye the comparative emptiness of that present moment for him, and this emptiness can terrify.

Sassall, except when involved in the actual treatment of patients, is the most impatient man I know. He is incapable of waiting and doing nothing. He is incapable of resting. He sleeps easily but, at heart, he welcomes being called out at night. He finds it extremely hard to accept as normal the normal content of a day, an hour, a minute. His passion for knowledge is a passion for constructive experience with which to so fill his time that subjectively it becomes comparable with the 'time' of those in anguish. It is of course an impossible aim: to construct, to relieve, to cure, to understand, to discover with the same intensity per minute as those in anguish are suffering. Sometimes the aim, as it were, releases Sassall; but mostly he is its slave.

Unrealizable aims possess many men – all artists, for example. The special stress under which Sassall lives is the result of his isolation and his responsibility. He cannot, like artists, give himself up to his visions. He must remain observant, precise, patient,

attentive. And, at the same time, he must face alone all
the shocks and confusion which have led to the
aim. If he were working with colleagues he would never
ask them: What is the value of a moment? Nor
could any of them reply, if he did. But the question
would present itself far less persistently. Their
presence would automatically supply the professional
context in which the implications of medical cases are
strictly limited. As it is, the implications for Sassall
can be almost limitless. What is the value of a moment?　ᕗ

I said that the price which Sassall pays for the
achievement of his somewhat special position is that he
has to face more nakedly than many other doctors
the suffering of his patients and the sense of
his own inadequacy. I want now to examine his sense of
inadequacy.

There are occasions when any doctor may feel
helpless: faced with a tragic incurable disease; faced
with obstinacy and prejudice maintaining the very
situation which has created the illness or unhappiness;
faced with certain housing conditions; faced with
poverty.

On most such occasions Sassall is better placed than
the average. He cannot cure the incurable. But
because of his comparative intimacy with patients, and
because the relations of a patient are also likely to
be his patients, he is well placed to challenge family
obstinacy and prejudice. Likewise, because of
the hegemony he enjoys within his district, his views
tend to carry weight with housing committees,
national assistance officers, etc. He can intercede for his
patients on both a personal and a bureaucratic level.

He is probably more aware of making mistakes in
diagnosis and treatment than most doctors. This is not
because he makes more mistakes, but because he
counts as *mistakes* what many doctors would – perhaps
justifiably – call *unfortunate complications*. However,

to balance such self-criticism he has the satisfaction of his reputation which brings him 'difficult' cases from far outside his own area. He suffers the doubts and enjoys the reputation of a professional idealist.

Yet his sense of inadequacy does not arise from this – although it may sometimes be prompted by an exaggerated sense of failure concerning a particular case. His sense of inadequacy is larger than the professional.

Do his patients deserve the lives they lead, or do they deserve better? Are they what they could be or are they suffering continual diminution? Do they ever have the opportunity to develop the potentialities which he has observed in them at certain moments? Are there not some who secretly wish to live in a sense that is impossible given the conditions of their actual lives? And facing this impossibility do they not then secretly wish to die?

Sassall believes that adversity can temper character. But can their groping and sometimes blind unhappiness be called adversity?

What is the cause of boredom? Is boredom anything less than the sense of one's faculties slowly dying? Why do they have more virtues than talents? Who can deny that a culturally deprived community offers far fewer possibilities through sublimation than a culturally advanced one?

How much right have we to go on being always patient on behalf of others?

It is from questions such as these – and a hundred others that force their way up through the pauses between these questions – that the disquiet, which finally leads to Sassall's sense of inadequacy, first arises.

He argues with himself in an attempt to maintain his peace of mind. The foresters are not subject to the same frantic pressures as millions keeping up appearances in the suburbs. Families are less fragmented: appetites less insatiable: the standard of living of the foresters is lower but they have a greater sense of continuity. They may lack cultural opportunities

individually: but collectively they have their Parish
Council, their Moat Society, their Dart Teams,
etc. These all encourage a sense of community. There is
less loneliness in the Forest than in many cities.
They are, as they might answer themselves, as happy as
can be expected.

He refers the question back to his former self –
the surgeon, the doctor of stark emergency, who tried to
transform the foresters into Greek peasants. The
foresters have no illusions about life, he says, only a
small minority complain. Mostly they proceed with the
business of living undaunted. They do not allow
themselves – they cannot afford it – to be governed by
their sensibilities. The notion of endurance is
fundamentally far more important than happiness.

Abandoning his former self, Sassall now takes a
realistic view of the world we live in and its
brute indifference. It is the nature of this world that
good wishes and noble protests seldom mitigate between
the blow and the pain. For most of those who suffer,
there is no appeal. The Vietnamese villages are
burned alive though nine-tenths of the world condemns
the crime. Those who rot in prison serving inhuman
sentences which the jurists of the world declare
unjust, rot nevertheless. Most crying wrongs cry until
there are no more victims to suffer them. When
once the blow is aimed at a man, little can
come between it and the pain. There is a strict frontier
between moral examples and the use of force.
Once pushed over that frontier, survival depends upon
chance. All those who have never been pushed that
far are, by definition, fortunate and will question
the truth of the world's brute indifference. All who have
been forced across the frontier – even if they survive
and return – recognize different functions, different
substances in the most basic materials – in metal, wood,
earth, stone, as also in the human mind and body.
Do not become too subtle. The privilege of being subtle

is the distinction between the fortunate and the unfortunate.

Yet however he argues, the disquieting questions return. And the harder he works, the more insistently they are posed. Whenever he makes an effort to recognize a patient, he is forced to recognize his or her undeveloped potentiality. Indeed in the case of the young or early-middle-aged it is often this which prompts the appeal for help – like the cry of a passenger who suddenly realizes that the vehicle in which he is travelling is not even going near the destination he believed he was making for. If as a doctor he is concerned with the total personality of his patients and if he realizes, as he must, that a personality is never an entirely fixed entity, then he is bound to take note of what inhibits, deprives or diminishes it. It is the inwritten consequence of his approach.

He can argue that the foresters are in some respects fortunate compared to the majority of people in the world. But what is far more relevant to his own preoccupations is that he knows that the foresters are in almost all respects unfortunate compared to what they could be – given better education, better social services, better employment, better cultural opportunities, etc.

Talk of the 'bad old days' before the war can encourage a certain superficial belief in progress. But faced with the young – and the prospects before them – it is hard to maintain any such belief. Sassall is forced to acknowledge that, by his own standards, they are having to settle for a fifth best.

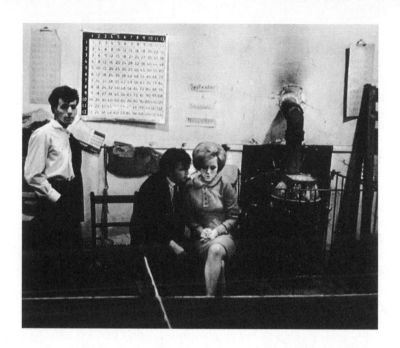

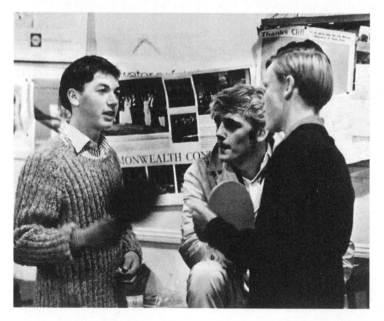

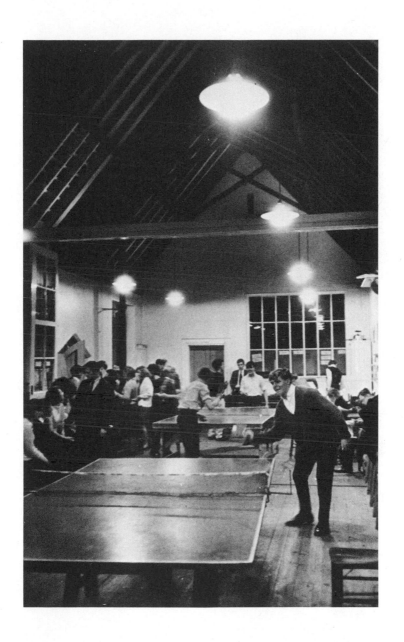

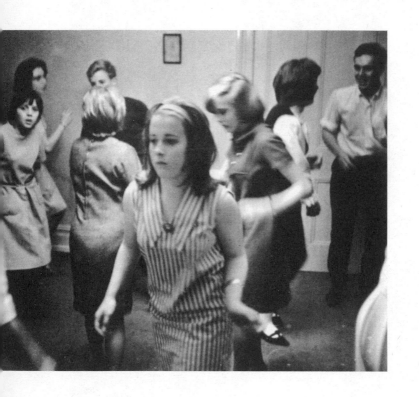

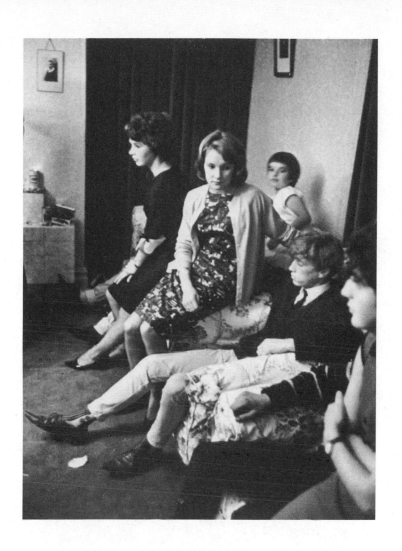

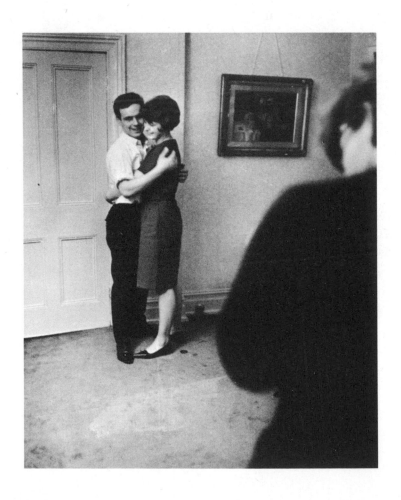

The situation by no means leaves him helpless. He can safeguard their health. Through the Parish Council he can urge improvements in the village. He can explain children to parents and vice versa. His word about a boy or a girl can carry some weight in the local schools. He can try to extend the meaning of sex for them. But the more he thinks of educating them – according to the demands of their very own minds and bodies before they have become resigned, before they accept life as they find it – the more he has to ask himself: by what right do I do this? It is not certain that it will make them socially happier. It is not what is expected or wanted of me. In the end he compromises – as the limitations of his energy would anyway force him to do; he helps in an individual problem, he suggests an answer here and an answer there, he tries to remove a fear without destroying the whole edifice of the morality of which it is part, he introduces the possibility of a hitherto unseen pleasure or satisfaction without extrapolating to the idea of a fundamentally different way of life.

I do not want to exaggerate Sassall's dilemma. It is one that many doctors and psychotherapists have to face: how far should one help a patient to accept conditions which are at least as unjust and wrong as the patient is sick? What makes it more acute for Sassall is his isolation, his closeness to his patients and a bitter paradox which we have not yet defined.

I believe that Sassall's disquiet is provoked, not by individual issues or cases because then all his attention is absorbed in 'feeling his way' and in reckoning how far he can go, but by the constant contrast between the general expectations of his patients and his own.

The average forester of over twenty-five expects, when healthy, little of life. (His extravagant expectation of fraternal recognition when ill is understandable precisely because the illness returns him to childhood, to a period before he had learned to abandon his hopes, and when these hopes could still be reasonably

satisfied within the family.) He expects to
maintain what he has – job, family, home. He expects to
continue to enjoy his pleasures – a cup of tea in
bed, Sunday newspapers, the pub at week-ends, an
occasional trip to the nearest city or to London, some
form of game, his jokes. His wife has her
equivalent pleasures. Both of them have fantasies which
are infinitely more resourceful and rich – perhaps
particularly the wife, who ages far faster. They also have
their opinions and their stories to tell, and these
may cover much wider ground. But what they expect in
their own situation in any foreseeable future is
very little: they may want more, they may believe they
have a right to more: but they have learned and
they have been brought up to settle for a minimum.
Life is like that, they say.

Their foreseen minimum is not purely economic: it is
not even principally economic: today the minimum
might include a car. It is above all an intellectual,
emotional and spiritual minimum. It almost empties of
content such concepts (expressed in no matter
what words) as Renewal, Sudden Change, Passion,
Delight, Tragedy, Understanding. It reduces
sex to a passing urge, effort to what is necessary in
order to maintain a *status quo*, love to kindness, comfort
to familiarity. It dismisses the efficacity of thought,
the power of unrecognized needs, the relevance
of history. It substitutes the notion of endurance for
that of experience, of relief for that of benefit.

This makes them, as Sassall is always observing,
tough, uncomplaining, modest, stoical. His respect for
them is genuine and deep. But it does not alter the
fact that his own expectations of life are diametrically
opposed to theirs.

It is necessary to emphasize here that we are talking of
generalized expectations rather than specific personal
ones. The question is philosophical rather than
immediately practical. Life is like that, the foresters say.
A man may be lucky and have everything he

wants, but the nature of life is such that this is bound to be an exception.

Unlike the foresters, Sassall expects the maximum from life. His aim is the Universal Man.
He would subscribe to Goethe's dictum that

Man knows himself only inasmuch as he knows the world. He knows the world only within himself, and he is aware of himself only within the world. Each new object, truly recognized, opens up a new organ within ourselves.

His appetite for knowledge is insatiable. He believes that the limits of knowledge, at any given stage, are temporary. Endurance for him is no more than a form of experience, and experience is, by definition, reflective. It may be that in certain respects he is prepared to settle for comparatively little – for an obscure country practice, for a quiet domestic life, for a game of golf as relaxation. (In fact on occasion he revolts even against this: four years ago he had himself accepted as the doctor and cameraman for an Antarctic expedition.) Within his outwardly circumscribed life, however, he is continually speculating about, extending and amending his awareness of what is possible. Partly this is the result of his theoretical reading of medicine, science and history; partly it is the result of his own clinical observations (he was, for example, observant enough to notice that Reserpine, given as a sedative, appeared also to cure chilblains and so might be useful in the treatment of gangrene). But above all it is the result of the cumulative effect of his imaginative 'proliferation' of himself in 'becoming' one patient after another.

We can now define the bitter paradox which provokes the disquiet Sassall feels at the contrast between himself and his patients and which can sometimes transform this disquiet into a sense of his own inadequacy.

He can never forget the contrast. He must ask: do

they deserve the lives they lead or do they deserve better? He must answer – disregarding what they themselves might reply – that they deserve better. In individual cases he must do all that he can to help them to live more fully. He must recognize that what he can do, if one considers the community as a whole, is absurdly inadequate. He must admit that what needs to be done is outside his brief as a doctor and beyond his power as an individual. Yet he must then face the fact that he needs this *situation as it is*: that, to some extent, he *chose* it. It is by virtue of the community's backwardness that he is able to practise as he does.

Their backwardness enables him to follow his cases through all their stages, grants him the power of his hegemony, encourages him to become the 'consciousness' of the district, allows him unusually promising conditions for achieving a 'fraternal' relationship with his patients, permits him to establish almost entirely on his own terms the local image of his profession. The position can be described more crudely. Sassall can strive towards the universal because his patients are underprivileged. ꙅ

From time to time Sassall becomes deeply depressed. The depression may last one, two or three months. He is not sure of the reason for these depressions. They could be organic in origin; conceivably they could be part of a still recurring but mostly hidden neurotic pattern established in childhood.

Yet if their origin is mysterious, their maintenance – if one may use the word – is revealing. By maintenance I mean the conscious material which his depressions requisition in order to justify and perpetuate themselves. With the fatal a-historical basis of our culture, we tend to overlook or ignore the historical content of neuroses or mental illness. Extreme examples in the distant past are sometimes admitted. One grants that there was a connection in the fourteenth century between the outbreaks of St Vitus's Dance and the suffering caused by the Hundred Years' War and the Plague. But do we appreciate, for example, how much Van Gogh's inner conflicts reflected the moral contradictions of the late nineteenth century? Vulnerability may have its own private causes, but it often reveals concisely what is wounding and damaging on a much larger scale.

Sassall's depressions are maintained by the material of the two problems we have just been examining: the suffering of his patients and his own sense of inadequacy. As reflected in his depression this material is distorted, but much truth remains even in the distortion.

He is working well. In a particularly complicated case he senses the number of disparate factors involved, and begins to trace the logic of their connection. He is planning some general improvement in his practice – the acquisition, say, of a cardiograph. He feels himself master of his own experience to date. The extent of what remains for him to do in the Forest is a confirmation of the rightness of his being there. He is always observant, but in this state of mind he notices far more than he can name or explain. Everything seems significant. And the stimulus of this so speeds up his selection and application of a myriad necessary routine responses and checks that he has time to speculate about what he is doing as he is doing it. He is working creatively.

The disillusion that he is about to suffer is likely to be triggered off by a minor setback with no serious consequences at all. A serious crisis could not have the same effect, for it would engage all his attention. As it is, he becomes slightly more self-conscious than usual about his responsibility. Something has not gone exactly as he would have liked for a patient. Yet the patient is quite unaware of it. He remains grateful or continues to grumble exactly as before. It is impossible for Sassall to tell him what he feels about the setback. Not for reasons of tact or medical etiquette. But because the patient would not understand and would still remain satisfied. Sassall is more sensitive to his patients' interests than the patient himself. He is more troubled by the setback than the patient will ever be inconvenienced by it. Thus Sassall's heightened awareness, instead of supplying him with new evidence and data – as it does when he is working well – suddenly draws attention to its own distinction. He has momentarily reached the threshold of mild paranoia. In the normal course of events the moment would pass with perhaps an ironic comment made to himself. But if at this moment he is unconsciously seeking a justification for being depressed, he can now begin to crush himself in the contradiction between his developed sensibility and the underprivileged life of his chosen patients. The challenges which have encouraged and confirmed him now seem proof of his presumption.

Guilty, he becomes increasingly susceptible to the suffering of others. This suffering, demanding its question about the value of the moment, reveals the comparative emptiness of his own life. To deny this, he tries, as we have seen, to compete with the intensity of suffering. He will work as hard as they suffer. His attitude to his work becomes obsessional.

Soon he is sufficiently depressed for his reactions to be slowed down and his power of concentration to have diminished. It seems to him that he can no longer meet the elementary demands of his practice. The challenge of what remains to be done – even the fabricated ethical basis of his obsession with work – suddenly seems to belong to another, vanished world. He believes that he cannot perform as a doctor on any level.

In fact he can and is probably still, at such moments, offering treatment which is better than the national G.P. average. But he can only partially overcome his conviction of inadequacy by admitting it. And

so, to those of his patients who are in a state to be able
to accept his confession, he admits his crisis.
He throws himself on the mercy of their tolerance.
He depends upon the fact that their demands are
minimal. The circle is complete. And, as often, the
completed circle is the seal of conscientious suffering.   Ɔ

Sassall is nevertheless a man doing what he wants. Or, to
be more accurate, a man pursuing what he wishes
to pursue. Sometimes the pursuit involves strain and
disappointment, but in itself it is his unique
source of satisfaction. Like an artist or like anybody else
who believes that his work justifies his life, Sassall – by
our society's miserable standards – is a fortunate man.

It is easy to criticize him. One can criticize him
for ignoring politics. If he is so concerned with the lives
of his patients – in a general as well as a medical
sense – why does he not see the necessity for political
action to improve or defend their lives?

One can criticize him for practising alone instead
of joining a group practice or working in a health centre.
Is he not an outdated nineteenth-century romantic with
his ideal of single personal responsibility? And in the
last analysis is not this ideal a form of paternalism?

He himself is aware of the implications of such
criticism. 'I sometimes wonder,' he says, 'how much of
me is the last of the old traditional country doctor
and how much of me is a doctor of the future. Can you
be both?'

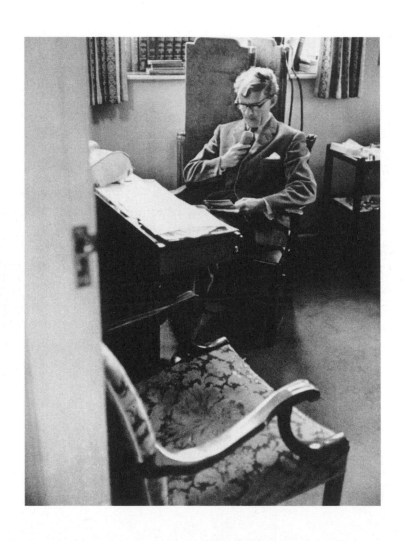

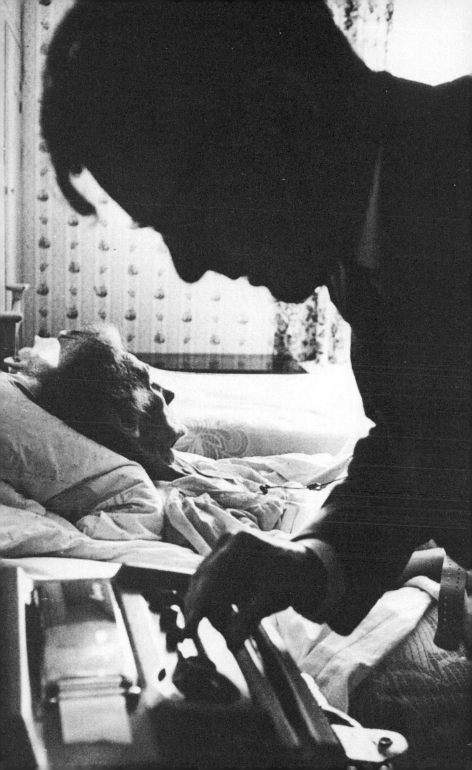

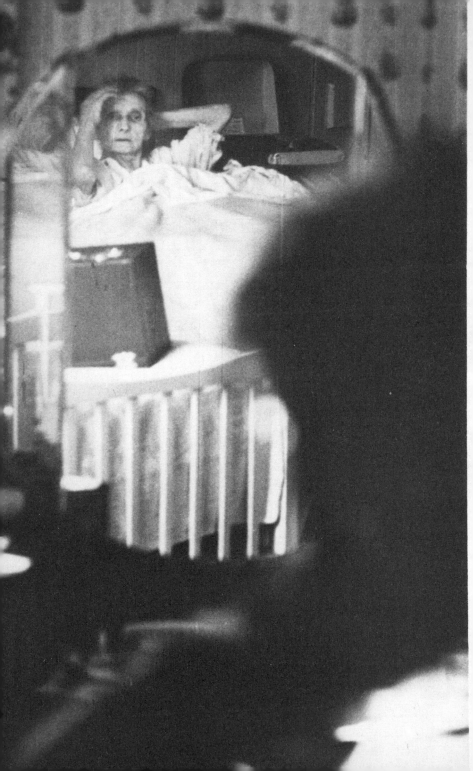

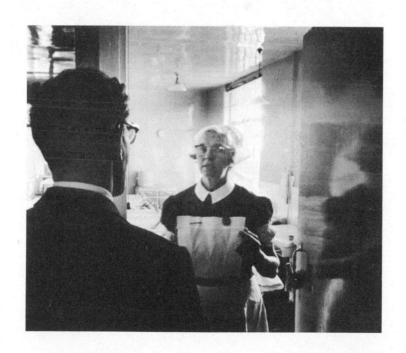

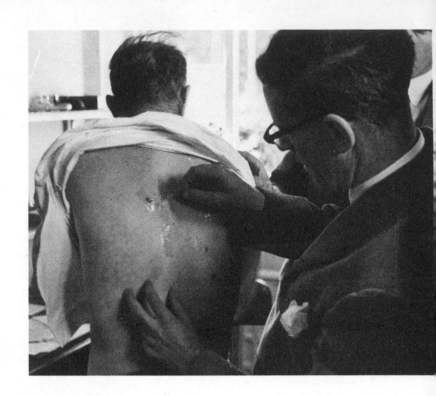

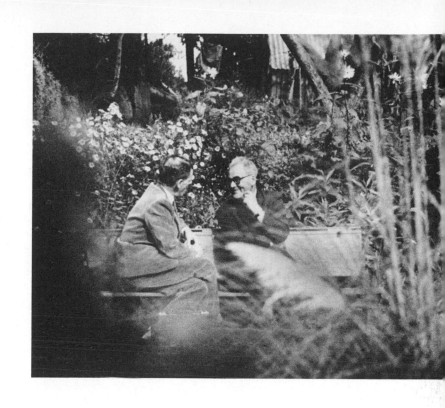

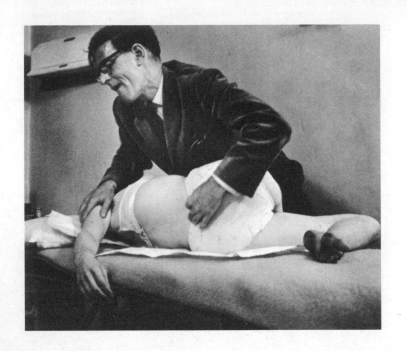

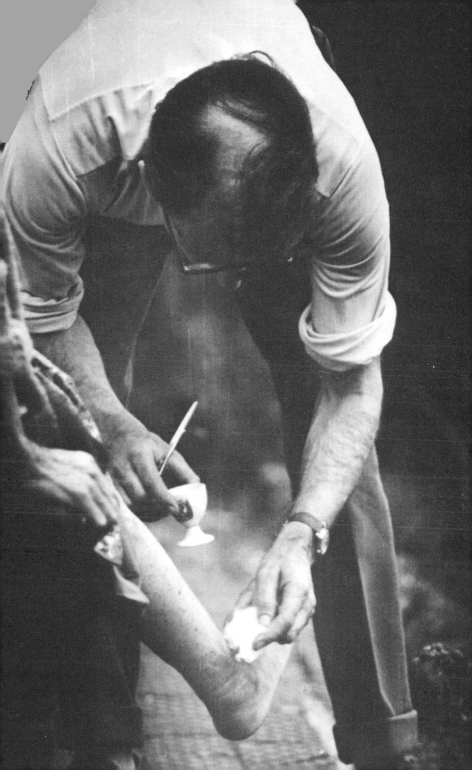

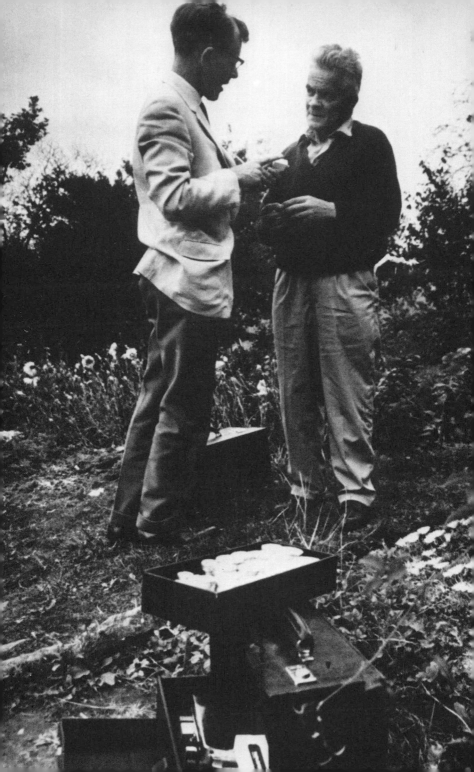

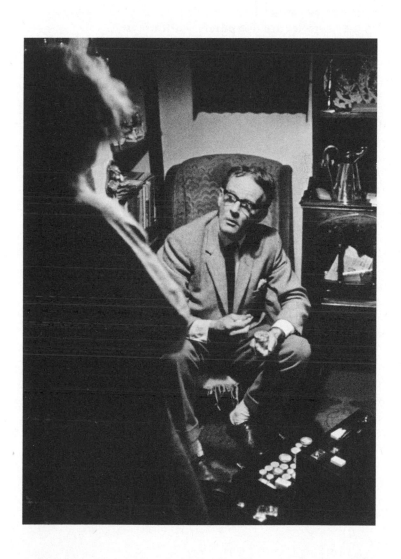

I wish I could write a conclusion to this essay, summing
up and evaluating what has been noticed. But I cannot.
It is beyond me to conclude this essay. I could end
with another story about Sassall and perhaps most
readers would then not notice the omission. It is to
reasoning that the poetic gives most of its famous licence.

However, it is perhaps more to the point to analyse
why the essay cannot be concluded – always assuming
that the obstacles are not purely within myself.

Nothing has in fact been concluded. Sassall, with the
cunning intuition that any fortunate man requires
today in order to go on working at what he believes in,
has established the situation he needs. Not without
cost, but on the whole satisfactorily. In it he is working.
He is working now at this moment as I write. He
may be prescribing a routine cure to a routine infection,
he may be listening, taking a few drops of blood
from a thumb, imagining himself to be the woman or
man opposite him, talking to a sales rep from
a drug firm, testing some urine, hoping to learn more,
learning more.

I have described something of the situation he has
established for himself: but finally this can only be
judged in relation to the work he does in it.
And I cannot evaluate that work as I could easily do if
he were a fictional character. In a certain sense,
fiction seems strangely simple now. In fiction one has
only got to *decide* that a character is, on balance,
admirable. Of course there remains the problem of
making him so: and the effect you achieve may be the
opposite of what you intended. But still – outcomes can
be decided. Whereas now I can decide nothing.

I am in the exactly opposite situation to the
autobiographer because he is even freer than the
novelist. He is his own subject and his own
chronicler. Nothing, nobody, not even a created
character can reproach him. What he omits, what he
distorts, what he invents – everything, at least by
the logic of the genre, is legitimate. Perhaps this is the

true attraction of autobiography: all the events
over which you had no control are at last subject to
your decision. Now, by contrast, I am entirely
at the mercy of realities I cannot encompass.

It is true that biographies, as distinct from
autobiographies, are also sometimes written about living
men and that these in their fashion come to a
conclusion. But the subjects of such biographies are
either famous or infamous. They are our future
prime ministers, or the foreign politicians of whom
we must take note. Both reader and writer before they
begin the book know why the book has been
written. It is because X is the famous X. And the story
naturally concludes when he has achieved
his present power, which is a form of apotheosis.

Sassall is not such a man.

And supposing he were dead? you might ask. But if
he were dead I would write a different essay. It
sounds absurd to say that a man's life is
utterly transformed by his death, but I mean for those
who knew him, or even knew of him. The simplest
confirmation of this is what happens when an artist dies.

The painting you saw last week when you assume
the painter was alive is not the same painting (although
it is the same canvas) you see this week when you
know that he is dead. From now on everybody will see
the painting you see this week. The painting of last
week has died with him. This may sound
excessively metaphysical. Yet it is not. It is simply the
result of our gift – or the necessity for us – of
abstract thought. Whilst the artist is alive, we see the
painting, although it is clearly finished, as part
of a work in progress. We see it as part of an unfinished
process. We can apply epithets to it such as:
promising, disappointing, unexpected. When the artist
is dead, the painting becomes part of a definitive
body of work. The artist made it. We are left with it.
What we can think or say about it changes. It can
no longer be addressed to the artist – not even to the

absent artist whom we have no reasonable chance of ever addressing; we can now only think and speak for ourselves. The subject for discussion is no longer his unknown intentions, his possible confusions, his hopes, his ability to be persuaded, his capacity for change: the subject now is what use we have for the work left us. Because he is dead, we become the protagonists.

It is the same in life. A man's death makes everything certain about him. Of course, secrets may die with him. And of course, a hundred years later somebody looking through some papers may discover a fact which throws a totally different light on his life and of which all the people who attended his funeral were ignorant. Death changes the facts qualitatively but not quantitatively. One does not know more facts about a man because he is dead. But what one already knows hardens and becomes definite. We cannot hope for ambiguities to be clarified, we cannot hope for further change, we cannot hope for more. We are now the protagonists and we have to make up our minds.

And so if Sassall were dead, I would have written an essay which risked far less speculation. Partly because I would have wanted to write a more precise memoir of him, to preserve his likeness. But also because when writing about him I would not have been aware – as I am now and have been every moment of writing – of the process of his life continuing – unfixed, mysterious, only half conscious of its own ends. If he were dead, I would conclude this essay as death concluded his life. Without sentimentality and without religious intimations, I would have wanted him to rest, at least on these final pages, in peace.

As it is, Sassall is alive and working, and my speculations have paralleled the process of his continuing life – anxious to see the maximum possible, but inevitably half-blind, like an owl in bright daylight. Too blind to see the conclusion for certain, aware only of the alternatives. ƍ

There is another factor which makes it almost impossible to conclude this essay. It is hard to write about it without making sweeping generalizations about our society and then having to justify these generalizations so that finally one is led too far from the subject in hand.

I must try to be simple. There are such things as national or social crises of such an order that they test all those who live through them. They are moments of truth in which, not everything, but a great deal is revealed about individuals, classes, institutions, leaders. The world at large does not usually appreciate or understand these revelations: but for all those who belong to the society or country in question their importance and meaning are quite clear. Even those who as a result of the crisis find themselves in total and lasting opposition to one another will nevertheless agree that what was revealed in the moment of truth was undeniable.

The word moments should not be taken too literally. The crisis may last for days, weeks, occasionally years. It was like this in Dublin in 1916.

> *MacDonagh and MacBride*
> *And Connolly and Pearse*
> *Now and in time to be,*
> *Whenever green is worn,*
> *Are changed, changed utterly:*
> *· A terrible beauty is born.**

It was like this in France in 1940 after the capitulation, in Budapest in 1956, in Algeria during the war of liberation, in Cuba when Castro landed for the second time in 1959.

If one were writing about a man who had lived through such a crisis and been illuminated by it, it would be much easier to see at least part of his life in

* W. B. Yeats's poem 'Easter 1916'.

perspective, to recognize his historic role. If one's
readers had lived through the same crisis, it would also
be very much easier for them to understand the
value ascribed to this role. To say to a Frenchman who
lived through the Occupation that X was in the
Resistance or was friendly to the Resistance, or that Y
was a *collaborateur*, is to say something about the
meaning of X's or Y's whole life.

Sassall has lived through no such crisis. He fought in
the war. But for Britain the Second World War
did not constitute a crisis of this order. In a crisis that
reveals and tests in the way I am suggesting,
every man has to choose for himself. By choosing for
himself he is then unequivocally committed with
all the others who have chosen likewise. It is as though
at a given moment each individual were waylaid
by the historical process of which he is a part and forced
to declare himself. In Britain in the Second World
War, we only had to endorse a choice which had been
officially made, and was daily justified officially,
on our behalf.

Since the war, during the last twenty years, we have
lived through a period which must be reckoned
as an exact and prolonged antithesis to a moment of
truth. We have exercised no choice at all. Certain
fundamental political decisions have been taken in our
name – without ever being presented to us as a
matter of choice. We have accepted them as inevitable or
with marginal protest. The Opposition in Parliament
is only an opposition about details: fundamentally
the two effective political parties are agreed. We have
been spared the obligation to commit ourselves to a
choice concerning any of the issues which occupy three-
quarters of the world as matters of life and death:
such issues as racial equality, the right to national and
economic independence, the ending of class exploitation,
the struggle for freedom (and survival) in a police state,
the abolition of famine, etc. We have our opinions,
but these count for little even as between ourselves.

Unaccustomed to choosing, unaccustomed to
witnessing the choices of others, we find
ourselves without a scale of standards for judging or
assessing one another. The only standard which
remains is that of personal liking – or its commercial
variant, which is Personality.

Many will say that this is our good fortune. I doubt it.
Our exemption from having to make choices has
been so far at the price of the constant deferment of
problems – basically economic ones – which vitally affect
our future. We will probably continue to defer
them until it is too late. Then we shall suffer our crisis
– perhaps in Sassall's lifetime.

I am aware of most of Sassall's opinions. I think I can
imagine how he might choose in any foreseeable
situation. But whether I imagine rightly or wrongly, or
whether all the possible situations are foreseeable
or not, the point is that any standards for assessing the
choice I believe he would make – the choice
which may confirm the purpose of his life – are
bound at this moment to be subjective, formulating
themselves as intimations rather than proper
measurements. They are bound to be subjective in this
way because in the present situation of exemption
and deferment it is only by a personal act of faith and
imagination that they can be kept alive at all.
Some pay lip-service to a set of objective standards by
which historic choices can be judged anywhere
in the world: but such people, with wild staring eyes at
the window, are all sheltering in various academies
of unfelt, dogmatic certainty. By contrast, my
intimations, which are felt, can as yet convince nobody
– and understandably so. We await the conclusion
of the long overture.   Ꝺ

Readers who have followed me thus far – to the furthest
outskirts of the subject – may now argue: *The future
has to be problematic: conclude by drawing up the
account to date: let it be an admittedly incomplete conclusion.*

But here we come to another difficulty. Sassall has practised medicine for twenty-five years. To date he must have treated well over 100,000 cases. This would seem a 'good' record. Would it be a less 'good' record if he had only treated 10,000? Supposing he is an intelligent but careless doctor – how much must he forfeit from his record for treating one case, ten cases, a hundred cases carelessly? Supposing that he is an intelligent and unusually dedicated doctor, how much must be added to his record? What would his bonus be?

Such accounting seems absurd. Then let us ask: What is the social value of a pain eased? What is the value of a life saved? How does the cure of a serious illness compare in value with one of the better poems of a minor poet? How does making a correct but extremely difficult diagnosis compare with painting a great canvas? Obviously the comparative method is equally absurd.

Should a doctor be judged professionally – by the consistent level of his professional skill? This would seem to make sense in the case of a surgeon, because his tasks, however complex, are limited. They have a beginning and an end and can be checked. A technique, however fine, is always within known bounds. It would be very much more difficult to judge a doctor like Sassall. However, I do not want to complicate the issue. Let us assume that the consistent level of Sassall's performance as a doctor can be measured as a technique. He can then be graded as a technician. Since with his technique he treats illness, and illness requires treatment, his grading as a technician should be able to determine the value of his work.

But could this satisfy us? The value of his capacity rather than the value of what he has really achieved?

Here I imagine readers interrupting: Of course it could not. But the limitation or absurdity of the answers is the result of the way you pose the questions. You cannot expect to evaluate a man's life's work as though it were stock in a warehouse. There is no scale of measurement possible.

It is true that my questions cannot be answered satisfactorily. But I was asking them to try to lead you to the point of realizing that we in our society do not know how to acknowledge, to measure the contribution of an ordinary working doctor. By measure I do not mean *calculate* according to a fixed scale, but, rather, *take the measure of*. It is not a question of comparing the doctor with the artist or with the airline pilot or with the lawyer or with the political stooge and then arranging them in a winning order. It is a question of comparing them so that in the light of the other examples we can better appreciate what the doctor is (or is not) doing.

When we hear of a team of doctors or biochemists discovering a new cure, we can acknowledge their achievement easily. A new cure contributes to 'the advance of medicine'. The acknowledgement is easy because the promise of the discovery remains abstract. It can be subsumed under 'science' or 'progress'.

It is a very different matter when we imaginatively try to take the measure of a man doing no more and no less than easing – and occasionally saving – the lives of a few thousand of our contemporaries. Naturally we count it, in principle, a good thing. But fully to take the measure of it, we have to come to some conclusion about the value of these lives to us now.

The doctor is a popular hero: you have only to consider how frequently and easily he is presented as such on television. If his training were not so long and expensive, every mother would be happy for her son to become a doctor. It is the most idealized of all the professions. Yet it is idealized abstractly. Some of the young who decide to become doctors are at first influenced by this ideal. But I would suggest that one of the fundamental reasons why so many doctors become cynical and disillusioned is precisely

because, when the abstract idealism has worn
thin, they are uncertain about the value of the actual
lives of the patients they are treating. This is not
because they are callous or personally inhuman: it is
because they live in and accept a society which
is incapable of knowing what a human life is worth.

It cannot afford to. If it did, it would either have to
dismiss this knowledge and with it dismiss all
its pretences to democracy and so become totalitarian: or
it would have to take account of this knowledge and
revolutionize itself. Either way it would be transformed.

Let me be quite clear. I do not claim to know what a
human life is worth. There can be no final or
personal answer – unless you are prepared to accept the
medieval religious one, surviving from the past.
The question is social. An individual cannot answer it *for
himself*. The answer resides within the totality of
relations which can exist within a certain social structure
at a certain time. Finally man's worth to himself is
expressed by his treatment of himself.

But since social development is dialectical and there is
always a contradiction between the existing social
relations and what is becoming possible, one
can sometimes perceive that the existing answer is
inadequate for questions raised by certain new
developments of activity or thought.

I have never forgotten a paragraph in an essay of
Gramsci's which I first read years ago. He wrote
the essay in prison in about 1930.

Thus the problem of what man is is always posed as
the problem of so-called 'human nature', or of
'man in general', the attempt to create a science of man – a
philosophy – whose point of departure is primarily
based on a 'unitary idea', on an abstraction designed to
contain all that is 'human'. But is 'humanity', as a reality
and as an idea, a point of departure – or a point of arrival?*

* Antonio Gramsci, *The Modern Prince and Other Writings*
(New York: International Publishers).

166

Is humanity as a reality and as an idea a point of departure or a point of arrival?

I do not claim to know what a human life is worth – the question cannot be answered by word but only by action, by the creation of a more human society.

All that I do know is that our present society wastes and, by the slow draining process of enforced hypocrisy, empties most of the lives which it does not destroy: and that, within its own terms, a doctor who has surpassed the stage of selling cures, either directly to the patient or through the agency of a state service, is unassessable.   Ɖ

The conclusion is inconclusive and simple. Sassall practises medicine. His practice perhaps corresponds a little to my description of it. Since we have as yet scarcely begun to establish a society which can assess his contribution socially, since we can only judge him, at best, by empirical standards of convenience, I can only end by quoting the logic by which he himself has to work, a logic which for all its stoicism has in it the seed of a great affirmative vision: 'Whenever I am reminded of death – and it happens every day – I think of my own, and this makes me try to work harder.'

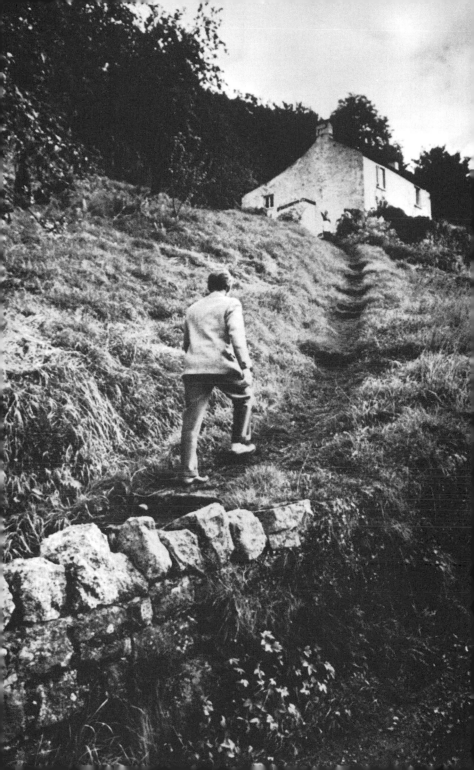

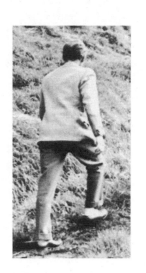